Overcoming the

DIETING DILEMMA

What to Do When the Diets Don't Do It

NEVA COYLE

BETHANY HOUSE PUBLISHERS
MINNEAPOLIS, MINNESOTA 55438

Copyright © 1991
Neva Coyle
All Rights Reserved

Published by Bethany House Publishers
A Ministry of Bethany Fellowship, Inc.
6820 Auto Club Road, Minneapolis, Minnesota 55438

Printed in the United States of America

Library of Congress Cataloging-in-Publication Data

Coyle, Neva, 1943–
    Overcoming the dieting dilemma / Neva Coyle.
       p.   cm.
    Includes bibliographical references and index.

    1. Reducing. 2. Obesity—Religious aspects—Christianity.
3. Reducing—Psychological aspects. I. Title.
RM222.2.C665   1991
613.2'5'019—dc20   91–24062

ISBN 1–55661–164–1 (hardcover)   CIP
ISBN 1–55661–232–X (trade paper)

There are few friends who are faithful and who stick by you in the days when you are the most difficult and unattractive.
I have such a friend.

Marieta

I dedicate this book to her.

"I will not sacrifice to the LORD my God burnt offerings that cost me nothing."
(2 Samuel 24:24)

I offer this book to the Lord.

NEVA COYLE is Founder of Overeaters Victorious and President of Neva Coyle Ministries. Her ministry is enhanced by her bestselling books, tapes, and teaching seminars. Neva and her husband make their home in California.

She may be contacted at:

P.O. Box 2330
Orange, CA 92669

Contents

1

The Dieting Dilemma

She was missing from the "Free to be Thin" class—which is a support group for those struggling with weight loss—and had been for several weeks. As I went over the calorie sheets from the members of my class that next week, I was surprised to see that one member, a friend of our "missing sheep," had written, "Neva, pray for Donna."

I sensed it was time to reach out. I phoned and left a message on Donna's answering machine, keeping it light but wanting her to know I was personally interested: "Missed you in class. Can you give me a call sometime this week?"

Days passed. No return call.

When she didn't show up the next week, I organized the class in small sharing groups, excused myself and found a phone. Again the answering machine frustrated me—but the tone of her taped message told me something that made me uneasy: Her voice sounded very *down*.

Something's wrong, I thought. Donna's past calorie sheets told me she'd hit a weight "plateau" and been stuck there for a long time—a real source of frustration for someone as diligent as Donna, who was precise and detailed in her food intake. She'd stayed cautiously within her calorie limit. Lately, I noticed, she had cut her intake even lower, and still her weekly weight record showed no loss. Thinking back, I remembered that Donna had been quieter, less cheerful during the last class she'd attended. Up till then, she'd been a bright encouragement to several others in the class during their times of struggle. Everyone liked her and we were encouraging her to hang in there until her weight began to drop again.

Two more casual monologues with Donna's answering machine got me nowhere. Finally, sensing that she was actually screening her calls, I took the plunge: "Donna, I'm very concerned about you. I'm going to drop by."

When Donna greeted me at her back door that evening, her face was tense. She was holding back tears.

"I can't see you now," she said politely.

"Please tell me what's wrong," I offered.

"I've been busy, that's all." Then came a string of pale excuses. But even before she'd finished, the tears had begun to spill down her cheeks. And finally—the truth: "I can't tell you how much I've dreaded seeing you."

As we settled at her kitchen table, I was already guessing at the painful "wedge" that stood between us.

"I have failed you, Neva," she said finally. With that came more tears. "I've failed the whole class. And I've failed my husband. I've even failed God. I'm not losing weight. In fact I'm *gaining*."

What followed was a profile of courage and endurance all from a woman who considered herself a "failure." She'd written down every calorie. No cheating. Exercised regularly. When the scale got stuck and would not drop, she cut out one meal a day, even though she got headaches and felt fatigued. She also prayed and dedicated her fasts to spending time with the Lord, not as a "bribe" but simply because she really was a good Christian woman. Eventually, futility and desperation had set in. Donna hesitated in her explanation, and looked away from me. "I've decided to try another weight group."

I did not want to burst her hopes, knowing as I did that a new group and a new diet was not her answer. So I asked casually, "Which group are you going to?"

"Well—" she hedged, "It's more like a clinic. They give shots. Kind of experimental. I know it sounds a little scary—but I'd do *anything* to get this weight off and keep it off. I've lost before and gained it all back again. And I just hate my life when I'm fat. I hate the way I look. I hate myself. When I'm overweight, I feel like I don't really have a life. . . ."

Donna did go to the clinic for those "weight-loss shots" despite the evidence I presented to her that there was no medical support for the clinic's claims, and despite my suspicions that they were placebos at best, potentially dangerous at worst. I've known so many men and women who have suffered disappointment, and even long-term physical harm, because the matter of weight has caused them so much frustration and grief that they have been willing to suspend their normally good judgment and try just about anything.

Up and Down—and Up

Maybe you too have been struggling with the "dieting dilemma." Like Donna—and countless other women and men—you may have tried one diet after another, one kind of pill or powdered drink after another. Maybe you've even tried some of the "miracle" discoveries and "scientific break-through" formulas. Some people lose weight for a time and get into a regular exercise program. Phase one seems to have worked: You look great, feel wonderful, and your self-esteem is soaring. If you're a Christian, you have a sense that by losing weight you've become a "good steward" of your body and that God is smiling at you—family, friends, and co-workers are sure smiling. You're a success!

And then . . . the scale, that old enemy, begins spitting some higher numbers at you again. The "thin clothes" you bought to reward yourself refuse to zip or button. Worst of all is the disappointment. But you fight back. Back to the diet, more strict with yourself than before. Back to exercising—more hours on the jogging machine, two aerobics classes instead of one. Or you try a different regimen altogether because the last one didn't work. And eventually, after a long struggle against the scale, you once again have success . . . for a time.

The cycle I'm describing is probably all too familiar to literally millions of men and women, both teenagers and adults. Many refer to it as "weight cycling" or "yo-yo-ing," an up-and-down-and-up pattern of loss and regain. For some it may be a matter of 15 to 25 annoying pounds that keep you from looking really good in a bathing suit. For others it may be more significant amounts—up to a hundred pounds or more—and the stakes may be much higher, involving serious health issues. Perhaps a doctor has even leveled an ultimatum: Lose, or else.

So many issues are wound into this matter of our weight, aren't they? Not only health and feeling comfortable with other people, but our self-image and worth, too. Perhaps it's for those reasons that some people get desperate when the weight won't come off and stay off—that many go into "phase two" of the weight-loss battle. Something inside tells you that you must commit to a life-long struggle against your body. It may be as simple as hopping from one of the latest "fad" diets to the next, from one diet book, plan, exercise program or clinic to another . . . endlessly. Or it may become much more serious, almost a gripping compulsion to lose, no matter what. For some that may mean severe calorie restriction, or bulimia, or more "acceptable" means, like surgery. At this point, you are willing to try *anything* to be slim again.

Whether you are feeling desperate to lose weight, or simply tired of trying and trying, I am writing to bring you good news and hope. There is a way to become free from the dieting dilemma. Years of great pain and personal struggle, counseling with many other fellow weight-strugglers, plus years of research have convinced me that the world of dieting and weight-loss—which has become a multi-billion-dollar industry—needs serious examination.

For me, the dieting dilemma led through many "victories" and "defeats" and close to disaster. Allow me a few moments to tell you how I know exactly what you're up against, and how I know that there is a way to overcome.

For me, there was great embarrassment added to personal fear and disappointment when, after losing a great deal of weight, the pounds began creeping back on. In 1978, I founded an organization called Overeaters Victorious. OV was and is a system of autonomous support groups that help, inspire, and teach biblical principles for living to the overeater, all for the purpose of leading men and women into a deeper relationship with Jesus Christ. A year later those principles became the basis for my first book, *Free to Be Thin,* which quickly became a bestseller. Quite literally, hundreds of thousands of people were finding help through the scriptural principles in that book.

The steps I so diligently taught others—and believe in to this day—are these:

1. God gives us clear-cut choices regarding how we are to live: Deuteronomy 29–30.
2. Rather than learn to diet, we learn to eat right as a matter of obedience: Romans 6:16; 1 Samuel 15:22.
3. God is speaking and we can hear Him—today: Proverbs 4:20–22.
4. Eating is a matter of stewardship: 2 Corinthians 5:10.
5. Obedience is a decision to live a life of higher quality, not according to mere legalism: Daniel 1:8; Jeremiah 7:23–24.
6. We need not be afraid of God-given guidelines and limitations: Psalm 119; Galatians 3.
7. God loves you and has a wonderful plan for your life, and He will show it to you: Colossians 1:9.
8. Our daily defeats and temporary failures need not affect our position in Christ: 1 Corinthians 1:30; Ephesians 1.
9. We really do need each other for support in life's important endeavors: Ecclesiastes 4.
10. Every work God starts, He completes: Philippians 1:6.

There is no question in my mind that these principles are *true*. I see now, however, that I had come to a wrong conclusion, based not so much on the Scriptures as on my own experience and on the values of our culture. I concluded that if you followed these principles religiously—making wise choices, learning discipline and self-control, getting support from fellow-strugglers—then you could pick a reasonable "goal weight," lose the pounds and keep them off from here to eternity. After all, that formula had worked for me—at first. And it was not that I condemned people like Donna; I was just sure that they had somehow missed some element of the formula, neglected to live by some scriptural principle, and so weight gain was a natural consequence. I never saw that I'd read into the Bible a promise that is not there: You need never be fat again. And I certainly did not see the implied judgment against overweight people: Being a well-disciplined person allowed you to enjoy the blessing of God (being thin), and disobedience left you outside the blessing (being fat).

It's true that if lack of self-control or eating to fill an emotional spiritual emptiness is causing you to overeat, and overeating is causing your weight-control problem, then the principles of OV will work for you. There are thousands who can attest to this. But I never knew the guilt and heartache my own words could produce in people who are *not* overeating; those who do everything right, but still cannot lose weight. I never knew, that is, until near-tragedy struck my own life.

"Success" Is Anyone Thinner Than Me

I started dieting seriously at the age of twenty-five. Though I was overweight, I was healthy, married to a man who loved and accepted me the way I was, and I had three healthy children, all of average weight. There was no other reason to diet except that I wanted to be thin: Appearance was the only reason. I was in for some big discoveries. I learned that the dieting world has a language, a set of rules and a culture that the non-dieter never experiences and, therefore, cannot understand.

For example, the *scale*. The bathroom scale became an essential part of my life. To be thin, I *must* own a personal scale. I went shopping and was overwhelmed by the choices: oval, round or square; colors to go with any decor; French provincial, butcher block, leather, cane, fur, fashion sable, marble, wicker, wood grain or nostalgia. I could choose a "hideaway" scale, or a portable model I could take with me on vacation. There were all-white models advertized as the perfect gift for a new bride. It was overwhelming, but I settled on an oval model with white plush covering.

Then began the daily battle with that luxuriously covered little machine. Often, I doubted its accuracy; sometimes I hated its accuracy. The white plush tyrant became a permanent part of my routine, weighing myself sometimes several times each day.

I was introduced also to the food scale. Non-dieters never weigh their food. I weighed every morsel. The very presence of that little Detecto scale in my kitchen made me feel guilty when my dinner serving of meat registered even a hair over three ounces. My little tool had turned on me. Instead of measuring my food, it measured my honesty.

Then began the research. I read all the diet books I could get my hands on, and bought every magazine that had a diet article featured on the cover. Research sent me scurrying to buy recommended gadgets and even more books. My calorie counters became a collection; I bought Bible study books having to do with weight loss. While attending a study group based on one of these books, I was stabbed with pain when the leader said, with all the disdain she could possibly show, she'd once been as big as a size 14. I was, in fact, paying quite a bit to *be* a size 14.

By this time, my whole mentality toward food had changed. Diet foods became a way of life for me, eating into an already-strained grocery budget. The sale of diet foods rose at a 10 percent annual rate between 1960 and 1980, amounting then to nearly seven percent of all food sales in the U.S. I'm sure I was the major contributor to those sales. I ate cottage cheese, Rye Krisp, and Profile bread. I even counted individual grapes, never eating more than eight large or ten small ones. I *never* ate more than half a banana, and measured my cereal by the ounce. I cut away all visible fat from my meat, stopped frying foods, and learned to steam my vegetables. I weighed apples and oranges, and determined *never, never, never* to eat chips, French fries or mayonnaise again. I went with my family to the pizza parlor and ate salad while they enjoyed pizza, and drank tea while they had sundaes and shakes. On Thanksgiving, surrounded by a feasting family, I ate only white turkey meat and a light helping of unbuttered vegetables. *Never dessert.*

A little success was wonderful. But the moment I relaxed my efforts a little, up went the scale. I began exercising. Into the house came an exercycle, a rebounder, and a treadmill. I also joined an exercise gym. Faithfully each morning, I rolled away "cellulite"[1] and used the machines to tighten, trim and reshape. One morning when I went to exercise at my friendly neighborhood gym—which had accepted my yearly fee just the week before—the building was vacant. Packed up and gone! No notice, no referral, just a sign that said "closed."

When exercising failed to give me forever-weight-loss, I consulted several doctors, one of them a bariatrician. He understood my desire and need for weight loss and gave me pills. "They're covered in my fee," he explained, "you won't even need to stop by the drugstore on your way home."

Taking the rainbow-colored pills, I became high. I never ate, and never stopped talking. I lost the promised pound a day—but I also lost sleep and friends, and drove my family crazy. When I finally stopped taking them I slept for almost two weeks. And I got hungry.

Discouraged, I read the ads for "Slenderella," Gloria Marshall, and Vic Tanney with longing, but never went. I read the ads for magic powders and weight-loss pills to help you lose weight while asleep. I watched Jack LaLanne on TV, while sitting on the couch. I was burned out on dieting and weight loss.

No doubt many of you will recognize the emotional cycle I was on, which is much more painful than the up-and-down weight cycle. You give up—for a time. Then something new comes along, and your hope and resolve flood in again. *This time* you're going to lose it and keep it off.

For me, the new thing was a support group. I'd been missing the empathy of other people—that was it. Hope returned. I felt I'd found help at last. I was no longer alone. I dieted faithfully, began losing weight, and discovered that it was okay to lose a little—but lose too much and others felt threatened. When the weight struggle began again, I switched to Weight Watchers. A lecturer promised good looks and self-worth—when we got to be thin. But I needed renewed self-worth now—not later. And I wasn't interested in carrying apples in my purse, or taking a sack lunch to the State Fair so I wouldn't be tempted to eat a corn dog. I wanted to be a normal person. I started to go only to weigh-in, until I realized I could weigh-in at home for free. I quit the group—but did not leave behind the conviction that I must become thin in order to be happy.

Yes, I had entered the world of the dieter—the society for those deprived of normal living, the cult of men and women who feel guilty for being a different size. Diets and methods and groups came and went. It was just a matter of time until I found the right one.

Then I discovered weight loss by another method: surgery. I decided to have an intestinal bypass. I would no longer have to diet. I could eat like a normal person, and, more importantly, feel like an accepted, attractive person after all.

In effect, I did not lose very much weight. Unexpectedly, I found myself sick every six months, with blood clots, kidney stones and other conditions that could be life-threatening. In a year, I had to have my gall bladder removed. And for years after that I had diarrhea and so much intestinal gas that I could never eat at anyone's house or go out to dinner unless I could leave immediately afterward.

At that desperate point in my life, in 1978, I started Overeaters Victorious. I had cut down to 850 calories per day, and lost forty-five pounds in four months. I was thin! I was happy! But I was already sick, and didn't even realize it.

Ten years later, with an established ministry to overweight people, and with my book *Free to be Thin* climbing to the one-million mark in sales, my health had deteriorated. Emotionally, spiritually, and physically I was a wreck, experiencing a high level of pain most of the time. Gas would build high in my stomach until I had severe pain in my chest, under my arms, and beneath my collarbone. Eventually it would move into my lower abdomen, causing tight cramping. I was forced to spend hours in tubs of hot water to relieve the agony.

Tests, X rays, examinations, and endless interviews brought the shocking news: I was dying of malnutrition.

That couldn't be! I knew the basics of nutrition and followed them to the letter—as much as my 850 calories would allow. But, in fact, I'd become so sick I could eat nothing but vanilla wafers, ripe bananas, cream of wheat, and tapioca pudding. Neva Coyle, Founder and Director of Overeaters Victorious, author of *Free to Be Thin* and subsequent Bible studies dealing with dieting—this woman who had helped so many thousands *couldn't* be dying of malnutrition.

I lived in a daze of denial. Could I really *die* if I didn't have corrective surgery to reconnect the intestinal bypass? That was the prognosis. Couldn't I just take massive doses of Maalox and Tums?

I prayed. Friends prayed for me. I cried to the Lord. I also got a second medical opinion.

Unfortunately, the verdict was even worse this time. "The truth is, you are already in a downward spiral," the doctor warned. "Life will be increasingly painful. You *can* reverse the process—but you can't delay any longer. You can choose life, or keep going downhill, Neva. No one can make the decision for you."

Even now, there was only one big question: Would I gain back all the weight?

The doctor stared at me. "This is not a decision to be thin or fat, Neva. This is a decision to live or die. Either way, there will be consequences. But—yes, in all the cases I've read about, reversing intestinal bypass will cause the patient to regain weight. Possibly, you will regain all that you've lost, maybe even within the first six months."

He went on with some "encouraging" news—that I could exercise and tone and maybe not regain all the weight—but my mind was numb. *By Christmas of this year, I could be fat.* How many times had I looked at the calendar pages and thought, *By Christmas I could be thin*? My life, as I knew it, was ending.

It is impossible to describe the guilt and pain. I felt like nothing but a big disappointment to all those in OV for whom I was supposed to be the model of godly discipline. Somehow, though circumstances were beyond my control, I'd let them down. Would they forgive me?

In the end, of course, there was little choice about the actual surgery.

I told my doctor, "I will do it. I have no choice but to choose life. I don't want to die." I began to cry.

But while waiting for the surgery, my spirits plummeted. I wondered if God was finished with me. I couldn't see any purpose in the hard work, the pain. All I could see ahead was fat—and that was like living death. Where was God?

New Life—New Understanding

It is amazing how new purpose can emerge in utter darkness—that is, if we will allow God to give us His plan in exchange for our own.

The night before surgery, my surgeon came in and sat on my hospital bed. I didn't know until that moment, when he told me, that he was a Christian. "I know who you are, too," he said. "My wife has read your book. I've prayed about the surgery, and prayed for you. I know what this is going to cost you. I understand the emotional trauma you are facing. I am convinced that this surgery is in God's will for you and in His plan for your life. You are an overcomer. You're going to be fine."

When he left and I was alone in the dark, I didn't feel like an overcomer. I felt more like an innocent person condemned to the guillotine, with no one coming to save me in time. Standing at the hospital room window, I put my head down on my crossed arms and sobbed. I was frustrated, angry, wanting to fight—or to give up and die.

Yet somewhere, deep in my spirit, I knew: Fighting or dying—neither was the way of the overcomer. I knew I had to submit, and that submission had to come from my heart.

Just before daybreak, as I looked at the silhouettes of the palm trees against the dawn, I made up my heart, knowing that my life was not my own. I'd given myself to God as a child and I was not going to take charge now. I sat in silence, listening to my own breathing for several long minutes.

"All right, Father," I prayed, "whatever you take me through, I'm yours."

A gentle peace, like soft warm rain on leaves, touched my spirit. Not long after, the sun came over the distant mountains, beginning a new day.

"Just let me be aware of your presence," I continued to pray. "I need you to be so near me that when I wake up I will know you're there."

In the difficult days to come, after the surgery, I would face pain, both physical and emotional. But I clung to God's Word, and one verse kept coming to me in my daily times of stillness and rest with God. "I will perform that which concerns you" (Psalm 138:8).

God knew my heartache. He was at work; my part was to hang on. To my surprise, "hanging on" became far more than lying around waiting for something wonderful and blessed to happen. Over a period of time strength returned physically, spiritually, and emotionally. And some inner activity had begun, a new curiosity—about the whole world of diet and weight loss, the health and well-being of the overweight man or woman. I began to make some discoveries that shocked and infuriated me, even as they gave me new courage and determination. And freedom—freedom to be *me*, no matter what my size.

First, through months of research, evidence piled upon evidence showed me that not all overweight people are necessarily overeaters, as the popular thinking goes. You can eat normally, or even less than other people—and still have certain predetermined factors in your physical body that will make you disposed to being "overweight," according to the charts. So, in effect, there are factors at work over which you have no control, any more than you could choose the color of your eyes. Why weren't overweight people being told these things?

What the "Experts" Don't Tell You

Here are some of the serious findings that "experts" in the commercial diet and weight-loss industry were not telling us:

There is more evidence to connect a weight problem to genetics than to the food you eat.[2]

Each dieting experience results in the body adjusting itself in ways that makes losing more difficult.[3]

There is considerable evidence to confirm that obese persons do not eat more, and many times eat less than normal-weight persons.[4]

There seems to be a control system in our bodies that actually slips into gear to recall fat that has been lost.[5]

With very rare exceptions, none of the popular commercially available programs are based on current, scientific knowledge.[6]

Weight-loss surgeries are not as successful in the long-term as once promoted.[7]

We probably should be eating more, not less.[8]

Not all overweight people hate their bodies.[9]

Overweight women tend to be at a lower risk for osteoporosis than thin women.[10]

Some medical experts think that the negative health effects of being overweight have been overestimated.[11]

Medical researchers are now concluding, "If most dieters gain back the weight they have lost, we can no longer accept that it is the fault of the dieter."[12]

No more than *five percent* of those treated with diet or psychological therapy keep lost weight off over a five-year period.[13]

You can actually gain weight on less food.[14]

Eating for *health* instead of dieting for weight loss must become the basis for our eating.[15]

What "Life" Never Told You—and You Need to Know

Then I encountered my second level of discoveries. It began with facing my own judgments against myself, as my weight began to increase.

Back when I began my weight-loss saga, I'd been operating under the influence of some buried attitudes—and they seemed pretty ugly as I faced them now. For instance: All overweight people have a problem with eating too much and simply need to learn self-control. But I had come to the point where I was not eating enough to keep myself alive and had still been gaining weight.

I'd also believed that all an overweight man or woman must do to lose weight is to surrender this area to Christ and the fat would melt away. But now, I felt more surrendered than ever to His Lordship—and the weight was definitely returning.

Underneath it all, I had to face the mindset I had acquired so long ago: Overweight people are undisciplined, not as committed to Christ as they need to be. Also—and this was a really tough revelation—that overweight people were somehow second-class. I believe I picked up these messages at a young age from other people, observing how overweight people were viewed and treated.

But slowly, subtly, these attitudes permeated me and became my own. So when I began to view myself as overweight, all the judgments I'd picked up were turned against me: The person in the mirror was overweight, therefore she was automatically undisciplined, a good Christian only if she lost weight, less than fully alive—and a second-rate human being until the weight came off. How painful; how wrong.

Life never tells overweight people they are valuable as human beings while they're overweight. And others can project the judgment that we're less than spiritual if we carry extra pounds.

If you have labored under judgments like these, if you have fought with one diet or weight-loss program after another only to "lose" again and again, then you need the discoveries in this book to help you overcome your own dieting dilemma.

In the immediate chapters you will find some unhappy news about the diet and weight-loss industry. This was difficult to write, knowing how many men and women cling to this industry and all its claims for their hope. It's time to face the truth, however, that so much of the "help" offered is based on unfounded and even false claims, some of which can severely harm you. Some of the findings you read may stir you and even make you angry—but I hope the truth will ultimately set you free and give you new determination (and quite likely, save you a lot of money too!).

Beyond the disclosures—and this is most important—I want to set you on a new path of self-discovery, and help you plan a new *healthy* way of thinking, eating, playing, and living.

And for the Christian reader, there is ultimately the question of bringing your *life,* not just your weight, under the Lordship of Jesus Christ. Many of us have been caught in a mindset that says to God, "I can't possibly serve you right now, I have to solve this weight problem first." In our honest struggle to be "better stewards" of our bodies, it is possible that many of us unwittingly let the goal of losing weight sneak into first place, supplanting our most important goal, which is *to serve God at all times.* I know how subtly this can happen; it happened to me. But weight need not keep you back any longer from loving, and freely, joyously serving God. It need not keep you back from embracing Life.

Yes, there is a way out of the dieting dilemma. You can be free from obsession with food and diets. You can find purpose for your life apart from your weight. You can stop rejecting yourself and start feeling wonderful about yourself at any size. The way begins with learning the latest findings about being overweight and dieting, and continues with embracing new healthful eating and exercise habits—without the pressure to lose weight.

You can *overcome* your dieting dilemma and start living again. I am free. Free to be accountable only to God, free to eat and exercise for health and life and not for others. Finally, I am free to be myself. You can be free, too.

Notes on Chapter One

1. "Cellulite" is considered to be a myth by most of my sources. It seems that fat in women tends to dimple under the skin, which is thinner than men's skin. To get rid of "cellulite" one must lose weight all over.
2. Albert Stunkard, *New England Journal of Medicine* January 23, 1986.
   Science News 1989, 11–18:327.
   Journal of Obesity and Health, Francis M. Berg, editor, Route 2, Box 905, Hettinger, ND 58639.
   Mayo Clinic Nutrition Letter, Sept. 1990.
3. *International Obesity Newsletter* reviews.
4. Ibid.
5. Ibid.
6. C. Wayne Callaway, Associate Clinical Professor of Medicine, George Washington University, on behalf of the American Board of Nutrition.
7. Radical weight-loss methods (such as intestinal bypass surgery, stomach reduction surgery, gastric balloons, lipectomy or suctioning out fat deposits, appetite suppressant drugs, protein-sparing modified fasts) are recommended to be used only when being obese poses more of a health threat than the weight-loss method and only when a person's weight exceeds their desirable weight by 100%. It is also concluded that none of the above drastic methods offers a permanent solution and in some cases make matters worse with weight re-gain. *International Obesity Newsletter* reviews. *Journal of Obesity and Health,* Francis M. Berg, editor, Route 2, Box 905, Hettinger, ND 58639. *Mayo Clinic Nutrition Letter,* July 1990.
8. Weight loss by more moderate caloric restriction than very low-calorie diets may have a metabolic advantage, even though medically monitored over-the-counter liquid diets are expected to exceed $800 million in 1990. *American Journal of Clinical Nutrition* 1990, 51:167–172.
9. *Journal of Obesity and Health*, op. cit.
10. Ibid.

11. Paul Ernsberger and Paul Haskew, "Rethinking Obesity, An Alternative View of its Health Implications," *The Journal of Obesity and Weight Regulation,* (1987) vol. 6, no. 1, p.2.
12. C. Wayne Callaway, Associate Clinical Professor of Medicine at George Washington University, testifying before the March hearing of the U.S. House Subcommittee investigating the weight-loss industry.
13. Paul Ernsberger and Paul Haskew, op. cit.
14. Dieting reduces energy needs. With each losing weight/regain cycle it takes longer to lose and a shorter time to regain. *International Obesity Newsletter*, op. cit.
15. Ibid.

2

The Courage to "Rethink" Your Weight

If you've lived with the dieting dilemma—the down-up weight yo-yo-ing described in Chapter One—you're probably faced with another problem: the tendency to think of yourself, at some deep level, as a failure. In fact, that may be far from the truth. Like many others, you may be fighting one of the most courageous struggles of your life with little or no support, and continuing to battle even when the scale goes against you.

That was the case for both John and Teri.

John was a "star" in his weight-loss support group, one of the few men who attended regularly. When I first met him at a retreat, he'd lost more than a hundred pounds. He was elated, and the women in his group were proud of him, as was his wife. He displayed a pair of "fat" pants, and joked about keeping them in a corner of the closet "just in case." After a few months, when he started missing meetings, his wife made apologies when the group leader called to check on him. He was just so busy—with his children's soccer games, and being an officer of the PTA. She didn't say that he was also regaining weight.

Eventually, he went to a commercial weight-loss program, setting aside everything else in his life to concentrate on getting his weight down again. For a time he became their "star" too. But while he was losing, John would become very angry when he went bowling and everyone on his team would "chow down," while he sipped diet soda. With determination, he once more made it to his goal weight—but only temporarily. The last time I saw him he was wearing his "fat" pants again. He was one of the most discouraged people I'd ever seen.

Teri is in her late thirties, and has been on and off diets since her mother put her on her first diet at fifteen. Her mom ruthlessly monitored Teri's calories. With the buoyancy of a teenager, she quickly lost weight—65 pounds!—and was able to maintain her cheerleader figure for eight years, throughout high school and college.

When she married, however, and the first baby came along, she gained 35 pounds. By dieting, she lost it all and kept it off a whole year—until the next pregnancy when she gained it all again, plus more. After the birth, she continued to gain, with the dismal feeling that she was losing control of her body and her life.

From time to time, Teri went on another diet and would lose five pounds or so. But now the weight came back more easily. A graph of her weight chart over the last seven years looked like a stock market analysis—up and down, up and down. More recently, to her utter discouragement, it has been up.

Cultural Mistakes About Overweight People

Most of us accept the "truth" that being overweight is our *fault*—that it *is* a fault. There may even be superficial denial. "My parents let us eat anything we wanted as kids"; "My wife loved to cook fatty foods"; "My husband insisted I make big dinners, and it's just too tempting." Underneath the words, overweight people carry the burden of shame: We tell ourselves that we are defective somehow—we are to blame for being overweight *now,* whatever the first cause may be.

It's time to stop playing the blame game and take a look at new scientific and biological evidence.

It's possible—believe it or not—that in certain fundamental ways no one is "at fault" when it comes to the matter of a given individual's weight. It's time to shake off the old habits of blame and take an honest, courageous look at new discoveries.

One of those discoveries is in the area of human physiology. Researchers in the psychology and physiology of overweight have recently stated:

> Obesity is a disorder that, like venereal disease, is blamed upon the patient.[1]
> Obese people, like the physically handicapped, wear their "problem" for all to see at all times, and yet unlike those groups are held responsible for their condition. They can scarcely avoid interactions with others in which weight and eating behavior are an explicit topic of discussion, concern, and criticism, or a covert determinant of others' evaluations.[2]

And:

> The word *fatness* itself has a negative sound, somehow connoting weakness, laziness, lack of self-discipline. The word *fat* is seldom used even by health professionals, who substitute the word *obese*. A prevailing attitude is that the fat person could lose weight if he really wanted to; he doesn't because he is lacking in motivation and discipline. Society's negative feelings toward obesity are more seriously reflected in its attempted denial of such an entity ... television ads promoting products for weight reduction demonstrate only successes, never the failures.[3]

In this light, we need to take issue with the psychologist who says people are overweight because they are depressed.[4] Is it any wonder overweight people can *become* depressed? Combine the social pressure to be thin, the cultural belief that we are at fault, and our repeated attempts to lose weight—only to regain, which results in consuming guilt, overwhelming helplessness and defeat—and the fact that more overweight people are not on psychologists' couches may be more like a miracle!

We are a culture that has been trained to see "thin" as the ideal. Most of us have been trained to judge ourselves according to "ideal height and weight" charts. The fact that we have been trained to *judge* ourselves at all, constantly measuring ourselves against other people, may be the first great mistake we need to rectify if we are ever to become whole, free men and women in Christ.

Once a "blaming" and a "thin-is-the goal" mentality are established, we are ripe for the next step in our trapped mind-set: We are trained to think that we can always do something to change the factors that cause overweight.

For years we have thought in very simplistic terms about taking off pounds by controlling our eating and exercise. Now, living in a more "scientific" and "high-tech" era, we're told that we can change our metabolism, that is, alter the natural "set-point" of our body weight. Though this sounds scientific, it too is an example of oversimplifying the complex mechanism of our body. The idea of the set-point really comes from engineering, using as its model the home thermostat. This handy gadget is made so that you can set the temperature at a certain level, and though the room temperature may vary a few degrees, it comes back to the temperature at which the thermostat is set. Basically, that's the same idea behind the set-point for body weight—that *perhaps* people are biologically programmed to weigh a certain amount.

We have also accepted the medical and social mentality that overweight *always* leads to poor health, an impoverished romance and sex life, less respect from families and business associates. What's more, we have accepted the diagnosis that as Christians being overweight is a poor witness to God's glory.

No wonder overweight people feel that they are living in a cloud of confusion about themselves, about those they love who should be supportive, and about God's view of them.

Only now is it becoming clear: There are factors beyond the control of any individual that can result in being overweight and even, by cultural standards, obese. It's time to replace old theories with new evidence.

Factors Beyond Your Control

"I knew you when you were formed in the secret place. . . ." Does this mean that my God and Father knew before I was born that I would have a genetic tendency—a secret, coded right into the strands of DNA, determining not only my hair color, eye color, and height, but even my *weight*—that I would be larger than the cultural "norm"? If new scientific studies are to be believed, then it is true.

Many of us have wondered—at times, in the pit of discouragement—if we have been *fated to be fat*. In our thin-oriented society this seems a fate worse than death. We try so hard, with little success. Yet researchers are now telling us to begin unlocking the "whys" of our weight by taking a good look at our parents—that indeed, a predisposition to weight gain may be fixed in our genes.

In a joint study between the University of Pennsylvania and the *Psykologisk Institut* in Denmark, Dr. Albert Stunkard, director of Obesity Research, and his Danish colleague Dr. Thorkild Sorensen have revealed new findings. These noted researchers gathered data on the weight of more than 500 adults who had been adopted as infants, along with weight data from both their natural and adoptive parents. To their amazement there was a strong correlation between the children's weights and those of their *natural* parents. Surprisingly, Dr. Stunkard says, no relationship existed between the children's weights and those of their adoptive parents.[5] In a summary statement they say: "We conclude that genetic influences have an important role in determining human fatness in adults, whereas the family environment alone has no apparent effect."[6]

These researchers are not alone in their conclusions. Just as counselors are discovering that emotional problems need to be resolved in family *systems,* those who are conducting serious studies on weight and weight gain are now concluding that genetics can be a main factor in determining the number of pounds you may be made to carry.

Aside from genetics, the common process of aging and other "natural factors" play an important role in determining weight.

Getting older doesn't mean that you *have* to get fat, but for many there are reasons why "older" will mean a tendency toward becoming overweight. For some, again, there is a genetic pattern: Some of us will get thinner, just like Dad or Mom. Some, on the other hand, will get fatter with age, just like Mom and Dad. This will be noticeable especially with the approach of middle age.

Aging is only one factor. Lifestyle change is another. Some, who lead very physically active lives in high school and college and then go into careers that promote sedentary lifestyles, find that weight can become a significant issue in mid-life. Running and playing is replaced by sitting and relaxing. Sports are replaced by quieter pastimes for many of us. Too, a high school athlete's healthy appetite is one thing—to be a big eater who sits behind a desk all day is another.

At first glance, these *seem* to be activities about which we can make choices: As adults we could choose to eat less, exercise more. But the truth—the real, hard truth—is that when we become adults, the "other" circumstances of our lives can take over and seem to wrest control. It is true that we cannot, need not, *must not* develop a victim mentality and blame others. But to be fair to ourselves we must honestly assess whether giving top priority to others has been an important factor in weight gain.

Let's face it, losing weight takes tremendous focus, time and energy. A young, active woman may suddenly find herself at home while raising several small children through diapers, scrapes and fights, illnesses, school plays, music lessons, and sports activities. Many young mothers, suddenly struggling with weight, have complained, "Believe me, if I had the time to exercise—to do anything for me—I would." Likewise the man who works hard for eight hours, faces a grueling commute, then has to care for home, lawn, and kids who want attention: Where does he find the time and energy? Add genetics and aging factors and you are headed toward weight gain.

Women, of course, can have their weight influenced by yet another factor: childbearing.

We know there is a natural tendency to gain weight during pregnancy. For some women, the weight comes right off. For many others, however, it remains "a problem."

In the 1950's, the recommended or "allowable" weight gain during pregnancy was established between 16 and 20 pounds for "normal weight" women and a weight-loss diet with no recommended weight gain for overweight women. The emphasis on weight control during pregnancy changed, however, after studies revealed that women working to keep their own weight down tended to deliver lower-weight babies that had more health complications because of low birth-weights. More recently, weight-gain limits were revised to no more than 22 to 27 pounds of weight gain during pregnancy.[7]

Most women report that after their first pregnancy they retain an additional five or more pounds above their pre-pregnancy weight. Breastfeeding has been an important subject of study of post-birth weight gain, with results indicating that nursing babies may indeed help get rid of extra stored energy (fat) prepared by a woman's body for that specific purpose. Animal studies have shown that pregnancy *not* followed by nursing of the young almost always leaves the subject at a higher weight than pre-pregnancy weight. Current recommendations have included breastfeeding a baby for as long as possible, both for the baby's sake and for the sake of the mother.[8]

Overweight women who become pregnant, unfortunately, gain more weight than thin women. Yet, while the pregnancy gain of a smaller-sized woman has a direct bearing on the size of her baby, not so the overweight mother. In her case, it seems that being pregnant often increases her weight more than that of the baby.

Yes, pregnancy itself can have an effect on a woman's weight. Some women, like Teri, find they begin a cycle of adding pounds that are increasingly difficult or impossible to get off with each pregnancy. One side factor may be that more women are working outside the home and returning to work quickly, thus reducing lactating time and not letting their bodies naturally dispose of the excess weight. More commonly, women experience "hormonal" changes—what our mothers referred to when they tried to comfort us with the words, "You're not a girl anymore, you're a woman"—that may also affect weight gain. What makes it worse for many of us who have gained stubborn pounds with pregnancy is that we live next door to the woman with four kids—each weighing ten pounds at birth—who still wears a bikini and has no stretch marks!

In addition to these factors beyond our control, the great, tragic irony is that you and I may have contributed to our overweight by our own struggles to get thin. Doing our very best to be "good stewards" of our bodies, it's possible—in fact, more likely—that we have actually, unwittingly induced weight gain.

Diet-Induced Obesity

Nancy is a woman who says she has dieted herself "into oblivion." "I try to eat right—I *do* eat right over ninety percent of the time. Yet whenever I lose weight I seem to gain it back again—and even *more*."

Is Nancy so unusual? Studies show that she is, in fact, part of a heartbreaking trend.

The experienced dieter enters each new program with enthusiasm and confidence. Each time they diet they hope that this new attempt will result in permanent loss. But, in fact, the prognosis is not good for this person: The long-term dieter is quite likely transforming himself, unknowingly, into the worst candidate for weight loss. Increasing evidence shows that the body can adjust to each dieting experience in unhealthy ways that actually make losing *more* difficult.[9]

Consider the testimony of Ray, who represents countless men who have worked hard, again and again, to lose weight.

Ray says, "When I lost the weight, I was obsessed with the fear of putting it back on, so I literally did just about everything. I tried behavior modification, slowing down my eating habits and that kind of thing. When the pounds began to return, I actually fasted a couple days a week, just to try to keep weight off. Or I would eat six apples to try to feel full. I really got fanatic, and also very scared. I found that I was not in control. I even went to a hypnotist to try to stop eating altogether. That worked for about three days.

"After about a year and a half, I gained back 130 pounds. Believe me, I fought it. I fought hard. And I probably could have kept it off—somehow—but I never found out how."[10]

And so, people like Ray can continue their search and struggle, not knowing that with each diet their chances of permanent weight loss are *decreasing*.

Robert H. Eckel, M.D., an endocrinologist and Associate Professor of Medicine at the University of Colorado Health

Sciences Center, has now declared: "We've looked at [over-weight] people in the wrong way. Putting weight back on is not necessarily a discipline problem. It is more likely a metabolic phenomenon, involving a mechanism in the body's fat cells."

Dr. Eckel's studies have turned up revolutionary findings: Fat cells actually work to maintain their own expanded size. Therefore, while we are fighting to take fat off, our fat cells are working hard to store *more fat* than would the fat cells in the body of a lean person.

"This preferential storage action makes it much more difficult to keep weight off," Dr. Eckel has concluded. Moreover, *"the more times the weight is lost, the more difficult maintenance becomes. With every weight reduction, the body will operate more strenuously to replace the lost weight"*[11] (emphasis added).

Such revelations are being echoed around the research community.

F. M. Berg, editor of the *Journal of Obesity and Health,* writes: "The thrust [to reduce] is for the victims to 'cure' themselves, get into weight-loss programs, learn more about counting calories, cut down on those numbers—*even though most people fail. . . .*" Berg went on to suggest that perhaps the time had come to be much more cautious in advising overweight people to "get onto weight-loss plans, since results are so variable. *There is no evidence that repeatedly going on weight-loss programs—even the better ones, incorporating both exercise and diet—is the route to success. Recent weight-cycling reports, in fact, suggest the opposite"*[12] (emphasis added).

Berg has also reported the findings of studies that indicate that we dieters are facing an uphill battle, if living at an "ideal" weight is our goal. More studies are verifying two conclusions: First, with every weight-loss experience the weight will return quicker each time; second, taking the weight off again gets harder with each subsequent attempt. In short, the *more* we lose and the *more often* we lose, the faster weight will return and the more difficult to shed in our next attempt. This is the meaning and the heartbreak of the newly discovered syndrome now known as *diet-induced obesity.*

Another obesity researcher, Dr. Kelly Brownell of the University of Pennsylvania, says in regard to this weight recycling issue: "We found that what our patients were telling us was true." Again: The more Brownell's subjects lost, the more they regained.

The New Facts—and What They Mean to You

- Dieters can face real, physiological obstacles to losing weight.
- Dieting can actually alter the metabolic rate, causing fewer calories to be burned as fuel and more to be converted into fat.
- The physical body can actually fight against you to regain lost weight.
- The yo-yo syndrome—or weight cycling—is well-known to repeat dieters, who diet and lose weight, only to gain it all back when they return to normal eating, and may in fact gain back *more* than they lost.

These are the new discoveries we've touched on. There is more you need to know.

More new evidence suggests that the cycle-dieter loses weight primarily from muscle mass, while the weight gained back is usually in the form of fat. In effect, repeat dieters are often condemning themselves to life-long obesity.

Research indicates that the best advice for dieters may be to ignore the cliche, "If you don't succeed, try, try again."[13]

What does this mean to you and me? It's time to face the facts about the negligible success rates when it comes to treating our overweight condition by dieting. There is little evidence that obese persons necessarily eat more than others. Yet there is evidence to conclude that dieting has a negative effect on metabolism and that weight losses by *any* method are usually small and don't last.[14]

One out of every four people are on a diet at any given time, and over half of all adults in our culture are overweight—and for every 100 dieters, 95 will regain all their lost weight within one year.[15] Another researcher claims that *less than five percent* will be able to maintain a weight loss for longer than seven years.[16]

Maybe you know someone who falls into that fortunate five percent. It now seems likely that these folks became overweight because of depression-induced overeating, or just overeating because of carelessness. In that case, once they dealt with the factors contributing to overeating and reached their goal weight they have gone on successfully with a thin life. But you need to be aware that many have *not* found it that easy.

No question—it is highly important to deal with the spiritual and emotional factors that can contribute to overeating habits and to victory, *whether you remain fat or get thin.*

But it is time to become free from shame if you are among the majority of overweight people who are subject to physiological and other natural factors that have nothing to do with discipline, obedience, or commitment. Maybe for some of us it is time to affirm that our commitment to the Lord *is* strong, that we *are* self-disciplined, honest, organized, energetic people who have tried so hard to lose weight. If the new research is to be believed, maybe the problem is that we've tried too hard.

I know: The research I've cited in this chapter is as frightening as it is exonerating. As I learned these facts, I found myself, many days, in tears, numb, or with an overwhelming sense of futility and discouragement. But as time went on a new courage came. I *was* being faithful in my eating habits. I *was* doing my best. I did what I *could,* and released what I *couldn't* to God.

My intention is that you find the same freedom. The freedom to walk responsibly in food issues, to find the freedom to be yourself.

To help you begin, I'd like you to sit down now and do a personal inventory, using some of the material I have shared with you as a base. Take a few moments and write down your answers to the following questions:

- How do I feel about myself being overweight? Do I dislike myself? Hate myself? Feel ashamed?
- How many diets (for weight control) have I tried? List them.
- How much weight did I lose with each attempt?

- What happened to me during and after each one?
  Socially:
  Spiritually:
  Emotionally:

Is it possible, in light of insights from this chapter, that your weight-cycling experience is a result of other factors—*not* because you haven't tried hard enough, or because you haven't been "faithful enough" to Jesus—but because you have tried too hard?

Do you dare to believe the findings you've just read? If so, what does it mean to you that the weight you're carrying now may be part of your life permanently?[17]

Think these things through carefully before going on. What you read next may change your view of the world of dieting and weight loss for good.

Notes for Chapter Two

1. E. B. Astwood, *Endocrinology* (1962), 71:337.
2. Benjamin B. Wolman, Ph.D, *Depression and Obesity, Psychological Aspects of Obesity—a Handbook,* (1982), pp. 130–162.
   S. C. Wooley, and O. H. Wooley, *Obesity and Women, Vol I, A Closer Look at the Facts* (Women's Studies Int., 1979), pp. 2, 69–79.
   S. C. Wooley, O. H. Wooley, and S. R. Dyrenforth, *Obesity and Women, Vol. II, A Neglected Feminist Topic,* (Women's Studies Int., 1979), pp. 2, 81–92.
   S. C. Wooley, O. H. Wooley, and S. R. Dryenforth, *Theoretical, Practical and Social Issues in Behavioral Treatments of Obesity,* (Applied Behavior Analysis, 1979), pp. 12, 3–25.
3. C. A. Craft, *Body Image and Obesity,* (Nursing Clinics of North America, 1972), pp. 7, 677–685.
4. Benjamin B. Wolman, Ph.D., op. cit.
5. "McCall's Monthly Health Newsletter," *McCall's,* July 1986.
6. A. J. Stunkard, M.D., Thorkild Sorensen, I. A., Dr. Med., Craig Hanis, Ph.D., T. W. Teasdale, M.A., R. Chakraborty, Ph.D., W. J. Schull, Ph.D., and F. Schulsinger, Dr. Med., "An Adoption Study of Human Obesity," *The New England Journal of Medicine,* Jan. 23, 1986, vol. 314, pp. 193–197.
7. "How Much Weight Gain During Pregnancy?" *International Obesity Newsletter,* June 1987, p. 2.
8. "Breastfeeding Found Beneficial for Mother," *International Obesity Newsletter,* Dec. 1987, p. 3.
9. "Why Can't They Lose?" *International Obesity Newsletter* (Hettinger, N.D.: Healthy Living Institute), vol. 1, p. 25.
10. "Fat Chance in a Thin World," a *Nova* video.
11. "Obesity Tied to 'Hungry' Fat Cells," *Healthline,* June 1988, p. 12.
12. *International Obesity Newsletter,* Jan 1988.
13. "Dieting-Induced Obesity: A Hidden Hazard of Weight-cycling," *Environmental Nutrition,* Feb. 1987, vol. 10, p 2.

14. G. Terrance Wilson, Ph.D., *Obesity,* (W. B. Saunders).
15. "Fat Chance in a Thin World," ibid.
16. Robert H. Eckel, M.D., University of Colorado Health Sciences Center, *Healthline*, June 1988.
17. After answering the questions, you may want to go to your local video rental store and ask them for the *Nova* tape, "Fat Chance in a Thin World." If they don't have it, they can usually order it.

◇ **3** ◇

"Anything to Be Thin . . ."

Recently, our culture has seen a remarkable move toward health-consciousness. Without question, the trend toward better health awareness and personal health-care is a positive step. Greater attention to our health gives us not only physical well- being, but brings a higher quality to our enjoyment of life as well. In this context, better health—controlled diets for reasons like controlling high blood pressure, heart disease, cholesterol, diabetes and other common conditions—is part of living a better, longer life.

Into this movement toward health-consciousness, however, two big assumptions have crept, winding themselves like vines around the original, good reason for controlling our eating.

One is the assumption that being overweight necessarily means you will be in poor health, suffer an impoverished emotional and even sexual life, be stunted in personality growth, and a swarming host of terrible corollaries. The second is the assumption that, in order to live the best life, you must be physically beautiful, or achieve physical beauty by diet, exercise and/or cosmetics. The assumption that being overweight always leads to poor health is now being challenged by researchers, which we will discuss in a later chapter. And the "beauty is everything" mentality, pushed by both men's and women's magazines, and the diet industry, also needs serious scrutiny. Until we separate out the truth about what is essential for good health from what popular culture chooses as desirable in terms of superficial appearance, we are in great danger of falling victim to the harmful message that "thin is always in," and victims to the commercial industries that promise us happiness through a thin, appealing body. Unfortunately, we Christians are not immune from the effects of the world's messages to us.

As a result of the powerful messages we receive every day of our lives, I believe too many of us fall prey to the "I'll do *anything* to be thin" mentality. Men are by no means exempt from this mindset, though it seems that women are predominantly the ones who struggle against weight gain, and often to the great detriment of their physical, emotional, and spiritual health. As we'll see, however, both men and women can become susceptible, under the pressure to lose weight, to try methods of reduction that are, sadly, outright *frauds*.

The Pressure on Women

By age three, it has been shown, the female in our culture sees fat as bad and ugly. By age *nine,* four out of five have already been on a self-imposed diet to lose weight.[1] In the minds of little girls, who should be jumping rope and playing jacks, the fear of fat has already taken root.

In one study, involving 11,000 eighth- and tenth-grade students, approximately 61% of the girls reported that they had been on a diet to lose weight at some time within the past year. Eleven percent reported using diet pills or diet candies within the past year.[2] Remember—these are girls who are only thirteen to fifteen years old.

By high school, several studies reveal, almost *90%* of all girls questioned say they want to be thinner, regardless of their present body weight. Fat girls want to be thinner, normal weight girls do too, as do thin girls. As a result, many of these girls were starving themselves while working out as cheerleaders or majorettes. For some, the practice of starvation dieting becomes a way of life, and even though they may become emaciated and ill, they continue to see themselves as fat and ugly and the diet, as a way of life, goes on.

The majority of women diet by the time they graduate from high school, and a recent survey of Tufts University first-year women indicated that although 95% were at ideal body weight, 85% felt they should diet, and 60% were actually dieting.[3]

Regarding adult women in general, women are more likely than men to say they have been overweight.[4] Almost 50% report that they are presently overweight—despite hard statistics presented by the National Center for Health Statistics that conclude only 16% are actually 30% over desirable weight. Further, caucasian women are more likely than non-caucasians to declare themselves overweight, even though other scientific studies report that blacks and hispanics are more prone to being overweight.[5]

The Pressure on Men

While women may seek to lose weight in order to achieve a cultural ideal, men most often make weight-loss attempts for different reasons.

John Lennon, the former Beatle, has been described by biographer Albert Golman as being anorexic for most of his life, after hearing himself described as the "fat Beatle." The phrase apparently struck such a blow to his fragile ego that the wound never healed. He then starved himself to what he perceived as perfection.[6]

A more common reason for men to feel pressured to lose weight comes in the workplace.

Harry Gossett, author of the book *Fat Chance*, recalls losing weight to keep below the weight standards of the FBI. One day, having been weighed by a new boss right after lunch, he was reported to the Washington, D.C., headquarters for being one half-pound over the standard. He was rendered "unfit for duty" and was found guilty of an official "offense," punishable by oral reprimand the first time, up to a five-day suspension the second time, and as much as a fifteen-day suspension the third time.[7]

In 1988, Ed Christy of Bath Township, Michigan, was suspended from being a volunteer firefighter because he weighed 260 pounds.[8]

Ken, the director of a hotline ministry in the midwest, constantly diets to keep a "good image of control and responsibility." Paul has lost and regained weight many times over the last several years. He keeps going on diets to lose after each regain because he gets passed over for raises if he is at a high weight when his performance review time comes around.

The University of Pittsburgh's Graduate School of Business studied 1,200 of their MBA graduates and discovered tall men earn more than shorter men, but if the taller man is slim and the shorter man is fat, the difference is nearly doubled. Male graduates who are 20% or more overweight earn $4000 less than their normal-weight counterparts.[9]

Others cite pressure from doctors, though the pressure is not always accompanied by useful dieting information.

James suffers from hypertension and vascular problems, and goes "on a health kick" to appease his doctors, but when symptoms abate, he slips back to unhealthy food-and-fitness habits. Leonard recently went on a strict diet when his arteries became clogged with cholesterol and threatened his life.

Questionable Methods—Needy People

The burgeoning weight-loss industry shows just how much we will spend on diets and diet products. What is frightening, though, is the proliferating market for diet programs, diet "aids," and even fraudulent products. For those who feel such pressure to lose, who have adopted the "*must be thin*" mindset, this is not the time to throw caution to the wind. It is a time for cautious scrutiny.

When people feel a desperate need, they are sometimes willing to try anything. So it is that "easy and safe" ways to lose weight have a certain appeal to life-long weight strugglers.

A recent study, conducted by the Harris Polls for the U.S. Department of Health and Human Services, concluded a high percentage of Americans do or are willing to use questionable health-care treatments. It was also discovered that many who use acceptable health-care treatments supplement them with questionable treatments, and about 14 million of those surveyed have used multiple questionable treatments. The result: More than one million persons report harmful effects because of questionable treatments each year; what's worse, it is impossible to estimate cases and costs of *unreported* harmful effects.[10]

The current estimate is that, excluding weight-loss products, $2.24 billion is spent each year on such questionable products. While the poor and sick are at special risk, the study also revealed that neither education nor income level is a protection against questionable product use. In other words, vulnerable people exist at all income levels, every educational level, and in every city and town in our country. When we hurt we can become susceptible. Who among us doesn't want relief—whether from physical pain, or from the inner pressure to lose weight because of emotional and psychological hurts? We hurt socially, emotionally, and even spiritually because of our perception of being fat, and we believe that all we need to do to fix the pain is to get thin. We want the pain to go away, and because of this we can be more easily hooked by advertising claims, without stopping to question.

Questioning the Ads

You're fat, and you ought to do something about it.

Any quiet evening, sitting at home after a hard day's work, it happens. You can be watching the news or your favorite series; you can be tuned-in to AM or FM radio. The message will find you. Suddenly we are confronted with products being offered by shapely models or high-paid celebrities, and always with testimonies by successful "losers" who promise us that we too can be thin. And even though we could be of average size[11], the message is that you *will* be happier, healthier[12] once you buy into *this* plan or product.

Do we ever stop and ask about the information that is drastically missing from these ads? It's time we learned something about ourselves and our own emotional make-up— things that marketing and advertising executives know and bank on. And it's time that we adopted a solid, reasonable set of criteria on which to judge the ads and promises that try to hook us. It's time you and I had a base from which to judge all the claims being made by products and programs, indicators and warnings to look for when critiquing a weight-loss plan. The American Dietetic Association (ADA) gives us such a standard, based on solid, credible information.

Recently, Congress began a serious investigation into questionable practices and outright fraud in the diet and weight-loss industry. Under the guise of caring friends, weight-loss professionals, or physician-approved, whole franchised chains have spread and grown. And as they've spread, so have complaints and reported abuses, so much so that government has begun to intervene. Fortunately, the ADA has begun to act also, giving us the help and guidelines we need to sift through advertising hype, revealing that little is left once the promises are stripped away.

In her testimony before congressional subcommittee hearings concerning fraud in the diet industry, Nancy Wellman, Ph.D., and president of the ADA, asserted that a healthy weight-loss program should:

1. present and encourage a variety of foods;
2. be specifically individualized to fit a person's lifestyle and food preferences;
3. encourage intake of no less than 1,200 calories per day, because of the danger of losing lean muscle rather than fat;
4. advise moderate diet with regular exercise;
5. counsel in methods of simple behavior modification.

Beyond these simple, common-sense guidelines, there are other questions we should ask *before* we try one of the widely advertised products or plans. Questions like: Does this product do what it promises? Are there statistics to back these promises? Where are the scientific reports and studies? What are the credentials of those making the claims? We should insist on verification: How many people using this product have taken off weight and kept it off? For how long? In essence, what proof exists—other than celebrity or other paid testimonials—that if I follow this plan I'll be able to take the undesired weight off and keep it off?

Before we look at the products and programs themselves, which we will do in the next chapter, I believe it's just as important for us to look at their advertising messages—some of them selling "legitimate" programs, others now being investigated for fraudulence—and consider why it is we are drawn to their offers again and again.

Deception

Through marketing and advertising research, ad and marketing execs know that we, the buying public, will be moved to purchase something if we believe it can:

help us achieve personal *happiness*;
keep us safe, or free us from something we *fear*;
help us to *gratify* something we feel we've been *denied*;
help us achieve a higher status to *feel better about ourselves.*

The unifying factor in these motivators is an appeal to our *emotions,* not our *reason* or *intellect.* For the overweight person who may have suffered rejection, self-hatred, and loneliness, these appeals are strong. Because of our *emotional need* to be thin, we can become susceptible to programs that, scrutinized by scientific means, deliver little or nothing in terms of long-range weight loss.

Let's examine just a few of the major ads, and see what it is we're really being "sold."

"Lose All the Weight You Can for $89.00. . . ."

On the surface this looks so good, doesn't it? It appeals to our sense of hopelessness, the sense that we *can't* lose weight, with an offer of hope. Therein lies the emotional appeal. It also seems like a good "buy"—in fact, it's exactly the opposite of the appeal restaurants use! ("All you can eat, for $9.99.")

But here's what closer examination reveals. This ad only *suggests* that I *can* lose, and that I can really get my money's worth out of the deal. But that is not anything like a guarantee of success. Testifying before the congressional subcommittee, Donald McCulloch, President and CEO of Nutri/System, Inc., said, ". . . that particular phrase was chosen with great care. We thought that the phrase 'lose all you want' was harmful." He goes on to explain that the slogan was chosen with business advice, not medical or scientific input. It has been demonstrated, however, that if a person has 99 pounds to lose and does so at the recommended 1 to 1½ pounds per week, it could take *up to a year and a half* and *cost in excess of $3,000.*[13]

Nutri/System, under pressure from the government, admitted that "the $89 promise" really only covers an initial fee. Those who buy in at $89 quickly find themselves hung on an emotional decision—to drop out when all their weight does not come off (and feel like a failure), or continue on much more expensively toward hoped for (but not guaranteed) success.

The Weight-Loss Professionals

What does "professional" imply to us? To those who have tried several times to lose weight on their own and failed, it can strongly suggest that one only has to turn over the problem to the "professional" for special and personal attention, assuring success. That is the emotional appeal—but what does the phrase mean to the Diet Center executives who use it as their advertising motto?

In testimony before hearings on fraud, Allan N. Stewart, president and CEO of Diet Center, said, "The meaning is that we are 'professional' in our delivery of a safe and effective weight-loss program." Not satisfied with that reply, investigators questioned the term "professional" further, and Mr. Stewart admitted, "Our counselors . . . have been trained in the delivery of a well-documented program, and we believe that they are *professional in the delivery* of that program, and I think [professional] is a matter of interpretation" (emphasis added).

So the *"weight-loss* professionals" are not professional at all in weight-loss studies—which would include professional health, fitness, and nutritional training. Rather, they have been trained in the *delivery* of the program—that is, in *sales.* By their own admittance then, these are professional salespeople, and their program is the product. But does it work? Is it safe? Will you get what you hoped for, paid for?

When questioned further, Stewart admitted that the Diet Center has no idea how many dieters have been unsuccessful on their program. Apparently, no long-term care or attention has been paid to anyone in their "care," therefore no such information exists.

Physician's Weight-Loss

". . . a team of physicians, nurses, and certified weight-loss counselors" is promised in the promotional materials by this nationwide weight-loss business. The implied promise is that there is close supervision, in this case by *medical professionals* who are specially trained in weight-loss. This appeals to an emotional need to know we are cared for by sincere, safe, and knowledgeable caretakers. But is that really the case here?

By their own admission to the congressional investigators, Physician's Weight-Loss centers are visited by *one physician, one half-day* each week, and the physician is available only to clients who ask to see a doctor. In most cases, however, there is no direct medical supervision, contrary to what the promise implies. Physician's Weight-Loss also claims that every client is screened by a doctor before admittance into the program—but what does it mean to be "screened?" A complete physical examination? No, that comes when and if the client has completed the program. The many who drop out are never "screened."

Then there is the very serious question about the training of the physicians involved. Weight-loss and its effects on health is a complicated matter that requires cross-disciplinary training in several fields. It is not true that any doctor is suited to handle any specialized problem. You would not, for instance, seek the help of a podiatrist in handling a blood serum problem. Likewise, the overweight person should only trust the advice of a medical professional who has cross-disciplinary training.

So it's important to know: Are the physicians who check in on Physician's Weight-Loss centers specially trained? Their own Medical Director, Dr. Jerry Sutkamp says, "No . . . our physicians have no special training in nutrition, other than what they learn in medical school." This is tragic indeed, since the Association of American Medical Colleges has found that 60% of medical school graduates don't get adequate training in nutrition, and that leaves them without a basic understanding of the complicated physiological and psychological factors involved in addressing the needs of overweight people.[14]

Senator Ron Wyden, chairing the investigations, expressed a concern we all should have: "I see 'Physician's Weight-Loss' up there in bright lights, and that says you have got trained physicians. But when we inquire about the physicians . . . the medical schools say more than half of their graduates don't work in the nutrition area, nor do they have any appropriate or special training."

These are just three examples out of the many "revelations" resulting from close scrutiny of weight-loss advertising, its claims and promises. Examining these and countless other ads could well make you ask, "If it's just clever advertising, isn't that considered *fraud*?"

No, these folks are not fraudulent in the legal sense of the term. They are just selling their product or services by clever advertisers and marketers who carefully phrase ads and terminology to "sound" like promises, which upon careful examination actually *promise nothing*. The real question is: Is this another type of fraudulence—emotional fraud—that will never be defined legally?

In the meantime, *let the buyer beware* is still an excellent motto to live by. Those who are trying to "sell weight-loss" need to appeal to more than our emotions, and we must be on guard not to let fear, loneliness, or hopelessness motivate us, when no *proof* of long-term success is offered. Don't allow emotions to keep you hopping from one program and diet to another.

Real Fraud

Simply stated, *fraud* is something the seller knows will not deliver the results they promise. Fraud is claiming that a product has a successful history, is recommended by experts, or is a new discovery, when those statements are known to be untrue. Weight-loss fraud is the promotion of false or unproven body-reduction products or programs solely for profit and not for your health and well-being.

The truth is, anyone can be taken in by actual frauds, not just "gullible" people. Let's look at some of the proven frauds.

The Diet Patch[15]

Before this scam was shut down, the dieter could purchase a sixty-day supply of patches and diet drops to be placed on the pericardium–6 acupuncture point, two finger-breadths above the junction of the wrist and hand on the palm side of the arm. This product, costing $50, and described as "about as effective as snake oil on a band-aid," was marketed on television through the new "info-mercial" format—that is, on long commercials that look like and intentionally mimic talk-shows, on which paid actors testify to the wonders of a given product. The viewer is led to believe that these testimonials, and indeed the whole program, is a spontaneous, unsolicited endorsement of the product being pushed. Often, 800-numbers are flashed on the screen, with telemarketing operators standing by to take your order and credit card number. *Beware.*

In the case of the "diet patch," thousands were defrauded before the FDA, the states of Missouri, Iowa, Texas, California, and the U.S. Postal Service took action against the manufacturer for fraud.

Chinese Slimming Tea

Full-page newspaper ads across the country claimed that Cho Low Tea had kept the Chinese slim for centuries, that it reduced cholesterol, reduced water retention, and aided in the digestion of fatty foods. The Food and Drug Administration declared it a fraudulent product, and also charged that the newspapers carrying those advertisements were fully aware of that fact. As it turned out, the perpetrator of the scheme was also wanted in England and in Australia for the sale of nearly $7 million worth of the worthless "slimming tea." If that wasn't enough, it was later learned that there wasn't any such tea at all—no packets to deliver, no warehouses to ship them from. The whole plan was a scheme to bilk millions from the dieting public.

Cal-Ban 3000

These capsules contain guar gum and cost $29.95 for a three-week supply. Anderson Pharmacals claims this ingredient "surrounds and combines with the food you eat and acts as a barrier to absorption of calories in the small intestine, particularly those calories from fats and carbohydrates." In legal actions taken by the states of Iowa and Texas, as well as the U.S. Postal Service, the makers of Cal-Ban 3000 have been ordered to cease and desist from falsely representing that the ingestion of Cal-Ban 3000 will, among other claims, cause significant weight loss in virtually all users and prevent food from being converted into stored fat.

Dream Away

"Just take Dream Away before going to bed. You will wake up the next morning slimmer, trimmer, and looking better than you did before." That's what the ads said—the Federal Trade Commission's investigation report says otherwise: "Dream Away does not cause a loss of weight or fat at all, while sleeping, or in a short period of time. It does not cause weight-loss without dieting or exercise, and does not contribute to the weight-loss effects of dieting or exercising." The states of Missouri and California have joined the FTC in action against this fraudulent product.

The list, sadly, goes on and on:

Amerdream: "We will pay you $1,000 to lose weight."

Fat Magnet: This weight-loss pill "breaks into thousands of particles, each acting like a tiny magnet, attracting and trapping undigested fat particles many times its size."

Maxilite/Fat Blocker: "Flushes calories right out of the body."

Frances Berg, editor of *Obesity and Health* warns:

The voice of the quack is soothing, secretive, and seductive, smoothly pitched to charm money out of vulnerable women, men, teens and children.

Because of our First Amendment rights, con artists are free to give false testimony against science, medicine, and reason. Not surprisingly, they take full advantage of this freedom. Thus, it is naive to believe, as many do, that, "If it's in a book or magazine, it must be true." Or, "The government wouldn't let it be sold if it could be harmful." Or, "If it's expensive, it must be good."

The voice of the quack often succeeds in its seduction. Money flows so fast that federal and state investigators can't keep up.[16]

It is at the point where we become unhappy with ourselves that we become fair game, vulnerable to the quack's enticing promises.

In his testimony, Carl Peck, M.D., Director of the Center for Drug Evaluation and Research, told congressional investigators, "In the weight-loss product area, it is often difficult to draw a clear line between helpful products and fraudulent products. While there is no easy method, or magic food, or device to melt away fat, we know the surest way to reduce health fraud is to reduce consumer demand for the fraudulent products."

The Food and Drug Administration reports a tremendous increase in fraud and quackery each year. Weight-control fraud is one of the leaders in this increase. Even though the voice of the quack in weight control will not cease, what Francis Berg says is true: "Through education and effective action we can reduce its sweet seduction."

How do you and I learn to recognize a potential weight-loss fraud? From Carl Peck's testimony we get good advice:

1. Be aware:

Know that weight-loss fraud does exist. It is not always obviously fraudulent, but can be simply a misleading or unproven claim in advertising. Look for words as a tip for deception. *"Breakthrough, secret, exclusive, special, accidental discovery, doctor tested"* are not scientific words, and often appear in promotions for quack products. There are no breakthroughs or secrets in weight loss.

2. Be cautious:

Question when immediate, effortless, or guaranteed remarkable weight loss is promised. Listen for vaguely worded testimonials.

3. Be wary:

Don't trust health remedies sold door-to-door by ped-dlers, friends, neighbors, or self-proclaimed health advisors who sell their products at public lectures during travel from town to town, or with high-pressure sales tactics.

Be wary too of products claiming to be Government-approved. *Having a patent does not constitute evidence of safety and effectiveness.* If the promotion sounds too good to be true, it probably is.[17]

Both the National Council Against Health Fraud and the *Obesity and Health* newsletter report that some medical in-stitutions, universities, and professional associations have compromised their integrity by operating diet programs with-out adequate accountability systems, accepting research grants with obvious commercial ties, and have linked them-selves with questionable corporate schemes.[18]

4. Be responsible:

Quackery works primarily through deceptive advertising. We must be more responsible in our own education and de-velop a certain level of informed skepticism. We can no longer depend on governmental agencies to do all our think-ing for us. The Federal Trade Commission (FTC) is overbur-dened with investigations and legal actions against hucksters in every area of fraud and fair trade, and has experienced substantial losses in funding since 1986. Andrew J. Strenio, Jr., FTC commissioner, told the American Advertising Fed-eration's Conference on National Advertising Law and Busi-ness that the future direction of advertising regulation is at a "crossroads."

According to the congressional hearings on weight-loss fraud, the Food and Drug Administration is too slow in their processes to ban ingredients and harmful drugs, while some-times acting too quickly to approve others.

Some consumer watch-dog groups are spending their ef-forts on creating what many consider an unjustified fear of America's food supply and safety, while ignoring the dimin-ishing area of consumer protection in advertising.

From Now On

The next time you see a commercial or an advertisement for a weight-loss product or plan, do yourself a favor. Use the information I have given you, and judge the product or program for yourself. Realize that you have access only to the information the manufacturer wants you to have and the word of those paid to do the advertising. Learn to be skeptical, in a reasonable, responsible way.

It is up to us to be better consumers, demanding proof before we buy. (For further guidance on detecting unsafe weight-loss plans and products, see Appendix A.) In an upcoming chapter, we will take a closer look inside "legitimate" weight-loss programs and learn what investigators are starting to discover. But first, a look at the "do-it-yourself," home-remedy methods of weight loss—and some health dangers that may be sitting right on your kitchen shelf.

Notes on Chapter Three

1. E. B. Astwood, quoted by Dalma Hein, "Body Hate," *Ms. Magazine*, July/Aug. 1989.
2. David F. Williamson, Ph.D., Center for Chronic Disease Prevention and Health Promotion Centers for Disease Control, Public Health Service, Atlanta, Ga., in testimony before the Senate Subcommittee hearings on Juvenile Dieting, September 24, 1990.
3. William H. Dietz, M.D., Ph.D., Associate professor of pediatrics, Tufts University School of Medicine, and Director of Clinical Nutrition, Boston Floating Hospital, in testimony before the Senate Subcommittee hearings on Juvenile Dieting, Unsafe Over-the-counter Diet Products, September 24, 1990.
4. Louis Harris and Associates, "Health, Information and the Use of Questionable Treatments: A Study of the American Public," for the U.S. Department of Health and Human Services, September 1987.
5. "Ethnic Differences in Fat Patterning," *Journal of Obesity and Health,* Dec. 1988, p.5.
6. *NAAFA Newsletter*, vol. XVI, no. 2, Aug. 1988.
7. Harry Gossett, *Fat Chance,* (Independent Hill Press, 1986).
8. *NAAFA Newsletter*, vol. XVI, no. 4, Oct. 1988.
9. Francis M. Berg, "Slim Males Earn Bigger Paychecks," *International Obesity Newsletter,* vol. 2, no. 1, Jan. 1988.
10. Louis Harris and Associates, "Health, Information and the Use of Questionable Treatments: A Study of the American Public," for the U.S. Department of Health and Human Services, September 1987.
11. According to *International Obesity Newsletter,* the average American woman is five feet four inches, weighs 142 pounds, and wears a size 12–14 dress.
12. While we may wonder, we don't ask if the model was ever more than 30 to 45 pounds overweight, even though the newest information tells us that being overweight by that amount is not as dangerous as once thought. "A few experts now believe that risks of being a few pounds overweight have been exaggerated," Dr. Albert Stunkard,

"Fat Chance in a Thin World," a *Nova* Video presentation.

13. House of Representatives Subcommittee Hearing: "Deception and Fraud in the Diet Industry," May 7, 1990, p. 35.

14. "Deception and Fraud in the Diet Industry—Part II," House of Representatives Subcommittee hearing, p. 33.

15. This and the following information is from the *Journal of Obesity and Health*, Sept. 1990.

16. Francis M. Berg, *Obesity and Health* Newsletter, Sept. 1990.

17. Testimony before the Committee on Small Business, House of Representatives, "Deception and Fraud in the Diet Industry—Part II," Carl Peck, M.D., Director, Center for Drug Evaluation and Research.

18. *Obesity and Health* Newsletter News Release, Dec. 15, 1989.

◇ 4 ◇

Do-It-Yourself Diets

"I feel like I'm doomed to be 45 pounds overweight the rest of my life—no matter what new product I try," writes Kim.

"I'm a pastor, and I know people are expecting *me* to do something about my weight," Mike confides. "I'm 60 to 70 pounds overweight. I see these professional sports figures on TV, telling how they lost weight. I even tried the product they were selling.

"It was awful—every week in the pulpit I felt like I was on display. Sure it was great for a couple of months, when the first 15 or 20 pounds came off. But when I regained it all, you wouldn't believe the judging looks I had to face every week. And the critical comments my wife heard—'Couldn't stick with it, could he?' 'I hope he doesn't plan to preach on self-control any time soon.' I can't tell you how destructive these remarks were. And how big a failure I feel."

"We've tried everything," Martin and Carie, an overweight couple, report. "Every magazine article that has to do with dieting, we've read. And every crazy diet we hear about we try. Why can't either of us lose weight and keep it off?"

I hear these same stories and questions over and over from men and women, teenagers and adults.

In large part, their frustration comes from the great amount of misinformation about weight loss. "We are all conditioned by the tabloid ad that tells us losing 60 pounds and keeping it off is easy," says Francis Berg.

With so many trumped-up advertising claims, it's no surprise that do-it-yourself weight-loss plans are now a fact of everyday life, as common on grocery store shelves as peanut butter. It's a way of life these days to depend on products, powders, and publications to assist us in our efforts. These do-it-yourself plans—from powdered drinks to diet books—present "new breakthroughs," "new discoveries," and "scientific secrets." Like most other claims, however, few if any deliver all they claim: The regain rate is still ninety-five percent—and possibly even higher. Yet we keep buying them because we fail to ask three very simple questions: Is this effective? Is it safe? Can they prove their "success" claims?

Let's take a look at the world of do-it-yourself dieting.

"Drink Yourself Slim"

> Mix it, flavor it, blend it, beat it.
> Whip it, mousse it, chill it, heat it.
> Shake it, stir it, or even freeze it.
> But whatever you do, *drink,* don't eat it.

The powdered drink meal replacement ads make it seem so easy and simple. Just a glass or two a day of their powdered food-replacement, plus a sensible dinner, and all your cares melt away with the pounds.

Can we believe what we are being told and sold?

Ray Johnson, Assistant Attorney General of the state of Iowa, thinks not. In his testimony before the congressional hearings on Deception and Fraud in the Diet Industry he said:

> Testimonials seldom, if ever, represent the typical experience a consumer can expect from taking the [powdered drink] product. In one case, the testimonials used in a television commercial were from paid models from a local talent agency, who were told that if they could lose a certain amount of weight in thirty days, they would get the testimonial work and modeling exposure.
>
> Another testimonial was from an individual who had lost a substantial amount of weight—but the advertisement failed to disclose that the individual was also suffering from a serious illness that was more likely responsible for his weight loss.
>
> The most frequent problem we encounter with verification of the testimonials is the fact that these companies are simply unable or unwilling to provide sufficient

information to locate the individual giving the testimonial. We can only speculate as to what we would learn about the testimonial if we could locate the person.[1]

Among the information these ads will never tell is the very serious health problems these products can aggravate or even cause. Yes, they promise quick weight loss, but fail to warn of lean muscle loss or quickly regained weight once normal eating returns, as it must. They don't tell us that once we lose weight by their method, and regain it, the next attempt will be twice as hard.[2] And this is only a sampling of the "missing" information. Let's look at some specific products.

Slim-Fast promises, "Give us a week, and we'll take off the weight." They fail to say, however, that using this product does not promote changes in long-term eating habits, which is always the case in diet regulation, or that they were originally designed for those who need to lose fifty pounds or more.

Dyna-Trim, another powdered drink product, promises you can "lose yourself in the taste," but does not tell you that you could lose your health in the process. According to ADA standards, the Dyna-Trim program and most others like it, are considered semi-starvation diets. The ADA also warns that living at semi-starvation levels of caloric intake is now considered by many experts the prelude to bulimia—that is, it can actually *promote* binging and purging by lowering an individual's metabolism to the point that it can trigger depression, a precursor and major factor in food binges.[3]

The supermarket isn't the only marketplace for meal replacement weight-loss schemes. The "direct-marketing" strategy is also widely used. Products such as The Last Chance Diet, Slender-Now, The Cambridge Diet, Herbal Life and United Sciences of America (USA) have all exploited friendships and family ties to help sell their products.

While using a particular product or line of products, available through direct-marketing schemes or at the supermarket, may be convenient and simple, *none has proven to be effective in its promised goal—permanent weight loss.* Each of the programs clearly violates ADA guidelines referred to in Chapter Three. For long-term weight control to be healthy and successful, the individual must take an active part in food choices, meal planning, and lifestyle decisions: No consideration for these important success factors exists in mass-market product-oriented pushes.

If failure to account for individualized needs were not weakness enough, there are real health dangers in taking these products, which are only now coming to light.

Into the Danger Zone

One of the claims the powdered-drink products proudly trumpet is their low calorie content. And yet, it is *because* of this deficiency that a dieter will dip below the 1200 daily calorie minimum, which, according to C. Wayne Callaway, is a dangerous "trigger" to binging when normal eating resumes.

In effect, none of these plans promotes a moderate diet, but rather a drastic and unhealthy practice, known as very low calorie dieting (VLCD). These temporary drastic changes in a person's lifestyle are not behavior modification; they are dangerous intervention.[4]

Perhaps there are times when the use of meal replacements is appropriate, and used occasionally they won't harm you. The experts warn, however, that they demand careful supervision and are not for everyone. Meal replacements can be hazardous when not carefully used.[5] The question is: How many of the 20 million[6] users of such products will seek out "careful supervision?"

In 1990 alone, sales of "medically monitored" and over-the-counter liquid diets were expected to exceed $800 million. Sales of nonprescription meal replacement supplements will continue to increase, and one research firm predicts that by 1995 these combined products will corner over $1 billion of the weight-loss market.[7] Alarmingly, product promoters do not have to produce any success/failure statistics concerning their claims and promises—let alone studies to show long-term effects on the health of their consumers.

Read Your Weight Off

In the publishing industry, it's an "inside secret:" Certain books will sell perennially and among them are, ironically, both cookbooks and books promoting "new" diets. A buyer from a major book distributor says, "Give us a good cookbook, or a new diet book—it doesn't matter. We can sell it year after year."

I once heard a statement that if man is still here 2,000 years from now, archaeologists will dig up books—not about food production and preparation, but books about eating. How to eat, when to eat, why to eat, and why not to eat. We love those diet books. They have a mysterious appeal.

Change Your Metabolism Diets

"Scientific discoveries" have shown us how to "make yourself what you want to be." That certainly sounds hi-tech. We read, discuss, and quote these "discoveries" at parties and Bible studies—but rarely question the validity of the material or require evidence beyond testimonials that these things really work.

Books like *The Underburner's Diet* by Barbara Edelstein, *The Yo-Yo Diet* by Doreen Virtue, as well as *The Beverly Hills Diet* and *The Atkins Revolution* are only a few of the books containing information based solely on personal opinion, and inaccurate, faddish nutrition "principles," according to knowledgeable reviewers. Title after title fails to educate the reader in healthful food choices, and such books rarely produce the results they promote.[8] Some are actually harmful.

For instance, *The Rice Diet* should be *avoided* by those wanting to lose weight, says reviewer Arlene E. Hoffman, a registered dietician (R.D.). Despite the author's claim that this diet is "state-of-the-art" nutrition, offering a "safe, scientific method of permanent weight loss," in reality the Rice Diet is not safe or scientific, nor does it result in permanent weight loss.[9]

Lisa Harris, R.D., writing about *The Life Extension Weight-Loss Program* says, "It is not recommended. It is overly dependent on supplements, promotes few healthful eating habits, and contains many erroneous and inconsistent statements.[10]

Yet these books have their appeal in the minds of modern dieters, possibly for two reasons. First, we've been trained to think that science and technology have the answers to everything. Because science is in the ascendancy these days, we sometimes dismiss logic and disengage our ability to reason when conflicting reports are published, and we accept the one which seems the most complicated in its explanation or claim if it is purported to be a scientific approach. Second, we've been affected, even as Christians, by a modern philosophy—the "religion" of our present time that tells us, "You can be anything you want to be. All you have to do is want it bad enough, and work at it hard enough." Never mind the fact that this is both humanistic and materialistic "doctrine." In real life people with good goals regularly are thwarted by circumstances beyond their control.

I don't say, "Throw out science altogether." Let's not go to the other extreme, but let's stay balanced. Remember this simple rule: Science is helpful, but not when it's harmful. When anything touted under the name of science harms God's creation and His plan, we need to take another look at its claim. In point of fact, you can actually use the latest "scientific" discoveries to help you get thin—and actually end up fatter later. This is well-known to repeat dieters who have experienced the "yo-yo syndrome," only to be told they had failed or cheated or lied. Now, evidence suggests something far worse may be happening than simply regaining lost weight. During initial weight-loss, as we've noted, muscle mass is lost right along with fat. But when weight is regained, it's not in the form of muscle, but fat. The effect may be that repeat dieters can condemn themselves to life-long obesity, assisted in part by these new "scientific" products and approaches.

I am convinced that what today's experts are telling us is true: Many of us are still fat, not because we haven't tried hard enough, but because we've tried too hard.[11] It becomes all the more important for those of us who have lost and regained to use the common sense criteria, such as that given in the ADA guidelines, in the last chapter of this book, to judge even "scientific breakthroughs" and "new discoveries." Just because it carries the label of science does not mean it is effective, nor does it mean it is safe.

The "Newly Discovered Diet That Actually Burns Off Fat"

Numerous books and tabloid articles claim that food combinations will magically melt fat away. They give us the impression that our unwanted excess poundage is just like so many gas-soaked rags on a garage floor, ready to catch fire by some spontaneous combustion within the body. It's as if we're supposed to read these books, eat our food in carefully planned combinations, run to the full-length mirror and chant, "Burn, baby—*burn!*"

Yes, it's true these diets cause you to shed pounds—not because you're eating fruits and vegetables in a special combination, but simply because you're eating more of them and less of other things. Unfortunately, you are likely to experience some unpleasant side effects, like bloating, initial weight gain, headaches, muscle aches, fatigue, nausea, and diarrhea. And even though the authors of such books show no concern about dehydration, it is one of the greatest hazards of this kind of diet.

Ignoring the body's warning signals is not the only problem with such scientific-sounding books. The important role of calories is often ignored completely. The body's inability to digest two "concentrated foods" at once is widely claimed, even though there is no support from the larger scientific community. The best-selling book, *Fit for Life,* claims that "the digestion of food takes more energy than running, swimming or bike riding. In fact, there's nothing you can name that takes *more* energy than the digestion of food." Yet the nutritional experts report that while the specific dynamic action of digestion accounts for the burning of some calories, it is very small in comparison to energy expended for other activities.[12]

The worst part of it is this: Many of these diets actually flirt with your health. For example, *The Rice Diet* recommends a 700-calorie daily allowance, which the dieter is to try to exist on for as long as possible. Not only that, the author recommends skipping meals, such as breakfast, whenever desired. It's no wonder she cites that dizziness and fatigue are common, helpfully suggesting that the occasional cold feeling will pass if you put on an extra pair of socks. The editors of *Environmental Nutrition Newsletter* comment, "The Rice Diet does not constitute a sensible plan for weight reduction. It is a starvation diet that limits caloric intake to below-recommended levels and eliminates whole food groups. Feelings of dizziness and cold limbs are not the sign of a healthy diet."[13]

The appeal of many of these diets is the "natural and healthy" approach plus the intrigue of a new "scientific" discovery. But while it's true we lose weight on such diets, we may lose our good health as well. Saddest of all, we will regain the lost weight long before we regain our lost health.

Who Is Writing All These Diets Books?

Many of us still believe that if something is in print, it must be true. Most of us are unaware that there are totally unqualified people—like journalists, businessmen, real estate brokers, sociologists, nurses, movie stars, housewives and athletes—who are writing diet books based on personal experience or theory alone. Many of these authors have no formal academic background in nutrition and seldom include input from those who do. As a result, they are responsible for propagating a great deal of diet *misinformation* each year.[14]

With a few guidelines, you can protect yourself from these unsubstantiated and even deceptive books. A general rule of thumb: Look beyond the sensational hype to find good, basic, reliable nutrition advice.

Yes, do look for a book that:

- *follows the United States Dietary Guidelines*—high in complex carbohydrates, low in fat, and moderate in protein. This translates to lots of whole grains, fruits and vegetables, no more than six ounces of meat a day, and only low-fat or fat-free dairy products. High-fiber foods should be embraced gradually, but excessive salt, sugar, and alcohol should be discouraged.
- *encourages a variety of foods.* Few items should be taboo. Rather, smaller portions of a few high-calorie foods should be suggested as a way to cut calories.

- *promotes life-long changes* in eating, not just a two- or three-week "diet."
- *encourages a gradual approach* to new eating habits. Changes made too fast are doomed to fail. Better to change one thing at a time and make it last.
- *gives practical suggestions* for incorporating dietary changes into everyday life, including meal planning, shopping, preparation, eating out, and special occasions.
- *encourages regular exercise* to keep fit, and provides specifics on how to start slowly and keep motivated.
- *uses language that is easy to read and understand.* A good book doesn't get bogged down in technical detail, and it often provides a glossary of complicated terms.
- *provides scientific references* when research is cited.
- *advises the reader to see a physician* before making significant changes in his or her diet.

No, don't buy or read a book that:

- *promises to cure a disease.* Many conditions may be improved or controlled by diet; some might even be prevented or delayed. But none—except outright nutrient deficiencies—can be cured.
- *promises fast results.* A weight loss of more than two or three pounds a week is not fat, but water, or worse, lean muscle tissue. The weight is easily gained back as soon as the diet is liberalized or forsaken. Some research even suggests that lost lean weight may be gained back as fat!
- *emphasizes one or two food groups* to the exclusion of others. A good diet encourages eating a variety of foods.
- *promotes the idea that certain combinations of foods are harmful.* Healthy people can digest proteins, carbohydrates and fats at the same time with no problem. In fact, most foods are a natural combination of these components.
- *encourages megadoses of vitamins and minerals.* With a varied diet of 1400 calories or more, supplements shouldn't be necessary. At any rate, there are few instances in which anyone needs to take more than 100%

of the recommended daily allowance (RDA). Before doing so, they should see a physician. Unbalanced nutrient supplementation can interfere with the absorption and utilization of other nutrients and medications.

- *denigrates traditional medicine* and the need for scientific research, while promoting the "conspiracy theory," i.e., that the information in the book is being held from the public by the medical community.
- *advises readers to ignore side effects* resulting from the book's advice. Side effects should never be ignored.
- *relies on personal testimonials* instead of scientific evidence.[15]

Getting hold of reliable diet information is why I subscribe to a wonderfully informative and credible newsletter called *The Current Diet Review*, published and edited by Lisa Harris, a Registered Dietitian in southern California.

You and I read and believe fraudulent and unfounded diet books, not because we are stupid but because we are tired of being overweight. We want an answer once and for all.

And what about *this* book? Am *I* qualified to write a diet book? No. But I am qualified to speak to you about dieting. First, I'm a person who has struggled all her life to control weight. I have read every diet book I could and reviewed countless others. Having written a million-copy best-selling diet book did not keep me from eagerly reading newer, "more scientific" diet books when I started gaining weight again. I, too, hoped that someone would discover a "key ingredient" that I might have missed in writing the Overeaters Victorious program materials. As a minister of the gospel, who has founded and focused a ministry on the spiritual and emotional needs and sufferings of overweight Christians, I wanted to be sure I was offering the best. While continuing to research what the experts have studied and learned, I have come to depend on the research of leaders in the field of nutrition—not the faddists. Only when I turn to the professionals do I dare to quote, or to promote certain food choices and habit changes. (Please read the footnotes, endnotes, and references to find out for yourself if what I have written is verified by others.)

In summary, the many years I've spent in ministry to overweight people have helped me to discover that reading diet books and accumulating "diet smarts" does not protect anyone from weight regain. Remember, our goal is not only to *lose* weight, but to become healthier in the process of changing our eating habits.

Remember, too, that your health and well-being are not always the goals of those trying to sell you a product or book.

The "Info-mercial" Game

Diet info-mercials, in the form of "talk shows" and "investigative reports" abound on cable and independent channels. A viewer who tunes-in after a program begins might never see the brief disclaimer that the "program" is really a long commercial message. Instead the viewer will see people claiming to be doctors and health-care professionals interviewed in a talk show or "new show" format. These "experts" will claim that their diet program or miracle diet product is a "scientific breakthrough" that is "safe," "easy," and "risk free." Consumers have no yardstick to measure such claims, or to evaluate the credentials of these self-proclaimed "experts."[16] Because of the well-planned format and carefully written script, consumers can emotionally connect to the presentation in such a way that they think they are buying these products with the advice of a real doctor, instead of entering into an over-the-counter type of transaction, fraught with risks and potential disappointments. The "info-mercial" host invites the viewer to "join millions of others"— fostering a sense of belonging or inclusion, when in reality the viewer is not joining anything: You buy a product, and you are on your own.

Just Stop Being Hungry

When the books fail, and they do; when the products ordered through an 800-number disappoints, and they will— we tend to believe that we have failed, that somehow we didn't have what it takes to remain "faithful" or strong. We blame ourselves, add guilt to our frustration—then look for something else to try. Our search now includes the need to find relief from the guilt of failure *in addition* to the struggle to lose weight.

I can do this, we say to ourselves. *I am an adult. If I want to lose weight bad enough, I can do it. There must be something wrong with me.*

Some of us decide the answer is simply to stop being hungry. Unfortunately, there are also products that can help us do just that. We go to the local drugstore or supermarket, and "pill" ourselves full.

Diet pills are not a thing of the past. They are ever-present, and their ads are very persuasive. Dexatrim, Acutrim, The Grapefruit Pill Diet Plan, and a variety of other brands and generic "house" labels line the shelves of our supermarkets, drug centers and neighborhood grocery stores. The diet pill industry continues to get financially fat by promising to help us get thin, making huge profits from the widespread use of their products—despite dangers and lack of evidence that they are effective.

For example, in 1979 the Food and Drug Administration approved a drug called *phenylpropanolamine* (PPA) as a diet aid. Since then, pill makers have spent $40 million annually on advertising PPA diet products. The medical profession has engaged itself in a long and losing battle with regard to the FDA's conclusion that PPA is both safe and effective as an over-the-counter drug.[17] Some consumers have become victims, losing their health while using over-the-counter diet drugs. Sadly, some have even become casualties.

Noelle was a promising, beautiful, fun-loving young woman, who began abusing over-the-counter diet pills at the age of sixteen. Just before she was to be married, she died of cardiac arrest. During college her use of diet pills had accelerated to as much as eight to ten boxes each week. A wholesome girl, from a good home with good moral standards, had resorted to stealing Dexatrim and Acutrim on occasion and borrowing money from friends when possible to support her abuse.[18]

We have been warned that the risks of taking these readily available diet pills are cerebral hemorrhage, increased intercerebral pressure, nausea, vomiting, anxiety, palpitations, reversible renal failure, disorientation, psychotic behavior, strokes, and death.[19] Yet these pills are available not only to adults, but to children, *without restriction.* Noelle's father says passionately, "These stores have no more business selling these drugs to children than they have selling liquor to a minor."

It is reported that girls as young as ten are buying and sometimes stealing diet drugs, putting themselves at severe risk to health hazards.

It is alarming to know that the drug PPA outsells aspirin, acetaminophen and ibuprofin by a significant percentage each year. Yet experts report that the side effects are grossly under-reported and understated by manufacturers, ignored by consumers, and that the use of diet pills is not and never has been the state-of-the-art treatment for overweight. In fact, they state that the use of PPA may not only be ineffective for weight loss, but may in the long-term cause its users to gain more weight after they stop using the pills. Health professionals are now decrying the validity of manufacturers' "studies" on the safety and effectiveness of their own products.[20]

Do we have any regard for future effects and dangers? The evidence given in the 1990 hearings on diet products and fraud in the dieting industry is shocking and dismal. For too many of us, the pain of being overweight blocks out all sense of reason, and we choose to believe that diet pills might be harmful to one young girl—but they won't harm us. Even though it might not be effective for most, we hope that it will "do the trick" for us.

Why is it that we let ourselves buy fraudulent products, such as Enzo Caps,[21] and Slim-and-Trim, and dream of waking up one morning really soon looking thin and trim?

"Fillers" and "Blockers"

When all else fails, some of us turn to fiber drinks and "blockers," products like Fast-trim, Manna-trim and Orignine.[22] We swallow Fiber-full, Fiber-Rich, and Fiber-trim. We use "starch blockers" and "sugar blockers," or diet-aid candies and bars.

As with the purchase of diet pills, it is all too easy to develop an emotional/psychological "dependence" on a substance, especially in a culture that already seeks its answers too often in chemical dependency. In effect, *none* of the products that promise to "block" the absorption of sugar or starch are proven effective in weight loss. Nor are the chemically "filling" candies.

It is time we asked the question—not "what does this product promise to do for me?" but "what can this product do *to* me?"

A Word to the Wise

We are attracted to the do-it-yourself approach, many of us, because of a need for control and independence. For some, it is important to keep our struggle private and personal. Many of us have tried between a half-dozen and thirty of these "do-it-yourself" plans and self-help approaches, not realizing how many others have tried and failed, too.

The National Council Against Health Fraud works hard to warn an unsuspecting public about useless and fraudulent health practitioners and products. And still, many of us continue to be driven by the hope that each book we read, each new diet we try or pill regimen we begin, will enable us to lose weight—even if we have to give up leading a normal lifestyle.

It is time to stop being victimized by an advertising-oriented media blitz that pops into our living rooms and automobiles with claims that appeal to emotional responses deep within us. Their frequency and catchy wording carry a degree of accusation that rings an all too familiar chord with our own self-critical messages. *They are not telling us the truth.*

Up till now, we may have simply taken the recommendations of paid celebrities and believed the promises of tabloid-type ads and testimonials. But that was before. Now we have criteria by which to judge those products and plans. We are no longer uninformed. We have a trusted base from which to build and form our own opinions, and make wise, healthy decisions about our bodies.

No longer do we need to be lured by the magazines at the

check-out counter, touting "The New Year's Resolution Diet, The First-Real-Date-in-Two-Years Diet, The Wedding Day Diet, The Honeymoon Diet, the It-Can't-Be-Summer-I-Haven't-Lost-Any-Weight-Yet Diet, the Before-the-Baby Diet, the After-the-Baby Diet, the I-Can't-Cut-Off-My-Thighs-but-I-Can-Stop-Eating Diet, the Ten-Year-Reunion Diet, the I-Wish-I-Was-Her Diet, or the Last-Ditch Diet."[23]

And for those who have fought through one or more of the franchised diet programs, it's time to look at some of the government evidence that has recently come to light.

Notes on Chapter Four

1. "Deception and Fraud in the Diet Industry—Part I," hearing before the House of Representatives Subcommittee on Regulation, Business Opportunities, and Energy of the Committee on Small Business, Washington, D.C., March 26, 1990.
2. "Yo-yo Dieting," *Berkeley Medical Health Letter*, Jan. 1989.
3. Dr. Ansel Keyes, reporting on a starvation study done at the University of Minnesota during World War II—"Fat Chance in a Thin World," *Nova* Video.
4. The American Dietetic Association Pamphlet: *Weighty Issues/Evaluating Diets*, 1987.
5. Francis M. Berg, "VCLD Specialists Warn Against Hazards," *Journal of Obesity and Health Newsletter*, March 1990, p. 17.
6. Janet Steiger, Chairman, Federal Trade Commission, and Barry Cutler, Bureau of Consumer Protection, testifying before the House of Representatives Subcommittee on Regulation, Business Opportunities, and Energy of the Committee on Small Business, "Deception and Fraud in the Diet Industry—Part I," March 26, 1990.
7. Francis M. Berg, "Liquid Diet Boom," *Obesity and Health,* July 1990, p. 49.
8. Based on information from several issues of *The Current Diet Review*, Lisa Harris, R.D., editor.
9. Arlene Hoffman, R.D., "Five Decades Old and Still Going Strong—the Rice Diet Report," *Current Diet Review,* vol. 1, no. 4.
10. Lisa Harris, R.D., "Manipulating Your Metabolism, the Life Extension Weight-Loss Program," *Current Diet Review*, vol. 1, no 5.
11. "The Weight Cycling Project," *International Obesity Newsletter,* vol. 1, no. 11, Dec. 1987.
    Rudolph L. Leibel and Jules Hirsch, "Diminished Energy Requirements in Reduced-Obese Patients," *Metabolism*, vol. 33, no. 2, Feb. 1984.
    Yves Schutz, Ph.D., Thierry Bessard, M.D., and Reic Jequier, M.D., "Diet-induced Thermogenesis Measured

Over a Whole Day in Obese and Non-obese Women," *The American Journal of Clinical Nutrition,* Sept. 1984.

12. *Environmental Nutrition Newsletter,* reprint article: "The Rice Diet Report."

13. Ibid.

14. Examples:
    Ursula Weatherton, M.S., R.D., "The Yo-Yo Is a No-No," *The Current Diet Review,* vol. 4.4, p. 3.
    Janet K. Leader, M.P.H., R.D., "With Friends Like This . . ." *The Current Diet Review,* vol. 4.4, p. 5.
    Hartsough-MacNeill, R.D., "A Victory in the Food Fight," *The Current Diet Review,* vol. 4.5, p. 5.
    James J. Kennedy, Ph.D., diplomat of the American Board of Nutrition, and board member of the National Council Against Health Fraud, "The Maturation of the Hilton Head Metabolism Diet," *The Current Diet Review,* vol. 4.2, p. 1.

15. *Environmental Nutrition,* June 1988.

16. From the prepared statement of the Federal Trade Commission, delivered by Janet D. Steiger, Chairman, before the Subcommittee on Regulation, Business Opportunities, and Energy of the Committee on Small Business, U.S. House of Representatives, March 26, 1990.

17. Committee on small business, House of Representative, Senate Subcommittee hearing, "Juvenile Dieting, Unsafe Over-the-counter Diet Products," Sept. 24, 1990.

18. Testimony of Mr. Anthony Smith, State Center, Ia., (Noelle's father) before the Subcommittee on Regulation, Business Opportunities, and Energy of the Committee on Small Business, House of Representatives, Washington, D.C., "Juvenile Dieting, Unsafe Over-the-Counter Diet Products," and recent enforcement efforts by the Federal Trade Commission, Sept. 24, 1990.

19. Denise Bruner, M.D., testifying before the Senate Subcommittee hearing on "Juvenile Dieting, Unsafe Over-the-Counter Diet Products," Sept. 24, 1990.

20. Testimony of Thaddeus E. Prout, M.D., Assoc. Professor of Medicine, Johns Hopkins University School of Medicine, and Chairman, Department of Medicine, Greater Baltimore Medical Center before the Subcommittee on

Regulation, Business Opportunities, and Energy of the Committee on Small Business, House of Representatives, Washington, D.C., Sept. 24, 1990.

21. *International Obesity Newsletter,* Oct. 1987, p. 8.
22. Ibid.
23. From an ad for Nike cross-training shoes.

◇ 5 ◇

"We're Only Here to Help You"

In a recent issue of *Parade* magazine, teenagers were asked: Is it okay to be different? Sixteen-year-old Gilana's response was published in a later issue.

"What kind of question is that?" she asked. "I've lived my entire life with people reminding me that it *isn't* okay to be different, because it isn't okay to be 16 years old, five-feet six-inches tall, have beautiful hair and eyes—and to be *fat.* It isn't 'okay,' and it isn't fair."[1]

How many of us, no matter our age, know just how she feels? How many of us have been convinced by two cultural myths—first, that *fat* is our *fault,* and second, if we wanted to be thin badly enough we could be?

"I can't speak for all fat people," Gilana continued in her letter, "but I do know that I am not lazy about losing weight. I'm always in the midst of planning a diet. I've tried sensible diets, liquid diets, crash diets. . . . My life is a 'Catch–22.' I'm lonely and I don't have any friends because I'm fat, and then I eat because I'm lonely.

"I have dreams about what it would be like to be thin," she finished. "There is nothing I would not give to be thin."

In my fourteen years of ministering to overweight men, women, and teenagers, more than 10,000 have written or come to me for help. Many are ready to go beyond the self-help level of dieting and failure. Many have asked for help and guidance in selecting a weight-loss organization. Most of these good people have already endured enough emotional pain surviving an overweight adolescence. Most have experienced failure after failure, and show signs of self-hatred, lack of confidence, and almost always *guilt.* They blame themselves for being fat, and assume the blame for their dieting failure and weight regain. Spiritually, they consider themselves rebellious for eating a single piece of wedding cake or a small slice of pizza. They're sure that God is unhappy with them and that the only way to please Him is to lose weight once again, getting themselves and their weight "in control."

Most have already tried the do-it-yourself methods: over-the-counter diet pills and potions; the latest magazine diets; some have even resorted to laxative abuse and vomiting. I know that for many of these folks—and perhaps for you too— one more failure and the physical, emotional, and spiritual consequences could be devastating.

As a Christian, a counselor, a minister, I have had to ask: Where could I send any of these people and guarantee a reasonable chance of lasting weight-loss success? Do the major weight-loss organizations and clinics offer lasting help, or even the acceptance their advertising images project? I will share with you what I've learned, and you can decide for yourself.

No Proof

What is the best weight-loss program? What do their success/failure statistics show?

The answer is: There are no statistics to prove any of the claims made by the major weight-loss plans or organizations. No statistics, and no information.

Surely if these organizations are claiming they "succeed where diets fail you," and that you and I can "lose all the weight you want"—surely there must be records and charts from their many clients to prove that they can help you achieve permanent weight-loss.

In response to my probing, a professional researcher told me, "I'm sorry, but there are *no* stats. There is no evidence available to prove any real and lasting success."[2]

Again, we are back to the hazy-gray world of advertising and images.

As we saw in a previous chapter, say the term "weight loss" and at least a half-dozen slogans leap to mind. Physician's Weight-Loss Centers claim to be the only program supervised by trained physicians. The name and slogans are calculated to leave strong, *unspoken impressions* that this is the "clinic" physicians would choose (and so should you), and that the program is medically supervised. Jenny Craig is identified by the ad slogan, "Lose all the weight you can for a $129.00 service fee." Diet Center offers you attention by "weight-loss professionals." Nutri/System promises you can "lose all the weight you can for $89.00." Even Weight Watchers International now offers a quick-start and personal-choice program, promising a three- to five-pound loss the first week.

Earlier, we looked at the emotional appeal of these claims. Now it's time to look deeper to see how the supposed success of these programs holds up under the light of inquiry. Can they deliver long-term weight loss?

This question prompted the Small Business Committee of the U.S. House of Representatives to begin their recent investigation, which I've quoted earlier. What did they find?

The nature of their findings is revealed in the title of the hearings themselves: "Deception and Fraud in the Diet Industry." This is not what overweight people, eager to lose, want to hear. Ethically, however, the findings that follow are what I must share with you. Knowing the truth could save your health.

Across the Board

The committee's general findings tell us that the weight-loss industry is presently a $32 billion-a-year business, probably growing to $55 billion within the next three to four years. As an industry, the weight-loss business is largely *unregulated* and *unsupervised*. Until now, no one has checked on its success/failure rates, and no one is offering these statistics either.

Why? Because, across the board, success rates are very, very low: *Few keep lost weight off, even for one year.*[3] The committee's findings, of course, square with what the diet and nutritional experts have told us—that approximately 90 to 95% of all dieters regain their lost weight, plus more.[4]

Congressman Ron Wyden, chairman of the committee, opened the session with these startling findings:

Many products peddled in the commercial clinics are *untested,* with *little or no scientific proof of their safety or effectiveness.*

Most "counselors" and "specialists" in commercial diet clinics are under-trained lay people, operating *without any medical supervision.* There are *no minimum standards* for their qualifications.

"Most commercial clinics promise fast, safe, easy weight loss. Yet most experts agree that fast weight loss is dangerous in and of itself. Further, little research has been done to show what does and does not work for each individual, according to the Surgeon General's Report on Health and Nutrition[5] (emphasis added).

Wyden was quick to note the government's failure to protect the consumer from diet fraud:

... despite the burgeoning deception and anger, the previous Federal Trade Commission has let the consumer program crumble, while hucksters multiply.

In the name of promoting competition in health-care, the former head of the FTC fostered an environment that led to a "buyer beware" medical marketplace, in which the scam artists could claim virtually anything with impunity, and did.

His conclusion: "... the safety of most of the popular commercial weight-loss programs is seriously in question." That included products offered and required by major weight-loss programs, which are largely untested, unlabeled, and offer no proof at all that they actually help the individual.[6]

What Do They Deliver?

The following information is sad, if not shocking. It comes, not from critics of the diet programs, but from top corporate executives under oath. What did these top men and women say in response to questions about their own organization's claims of professionalism and success?

Allan N. Stewart, president and CEO of Diet Center, Inc., was asked a number of questions, including: What can the Diet Center program deliver when it claims to be the "weight-loss professionals?'' Does this mean that the program is delivered by health professionals—doctors, nurses, registered dietitians? Do they have professionally kept charts and records of weight-loss success?

Stewart's response, as we saw earlier, was: "The meaning of [the phrase 'weight-loss professionals'] is that we are professional in our delivery of a safe and effective weight-loss program.''

As it turns out, "professional in our delivery" means merely that they are staffed by professionally trained salespeople, not trained nutritional counselors. There is no professional health-tracking of the dieting individual.

A. Donald McCulloch, Jr., president and CEO of Nutri/System, Inc., was asked, as we noted: What does the Nutri/System promise "lose all the weight you can for $89" really mean? His answer:

> . . . that particular phrase was chosen with great care.
> We thought the phrase "lose all the weight you want"
> was harmful.[7]

More important than all the clever, if insubstantial, ad-phrasing is: Who has the best rate of success? Who has the worst rate? Will any of the weight-loss "professionals" tell us?

Investigator Wyden asked for success statistics from Charles E. Sekeres, president and CEO of Physician's Weight-Loss Centers. Sekeres' carefully worded reply was, "We're not statistically oriented."[8]

Wyden asked a similar direct question of the Diet Center's Allan Stewart: ". . . do you have statistics on what percentage of Diet Center clients have been unsuccessful on a weight-loss program?" Stewart, now unable to hedge, said, ". . . the answer is *no*.''

Wyden followed up by asking, "Do we have evidence of how many people actually complete the Diet Center program through maintenance—specific numbers and percentages?"

"No, Mr. Chairman, we do not," was Stewart's reply.

Again and again, the congressional investigators ran into the same roadblocks. Not one organization in the diet industry seems to be able to produce any statistics to support their media images that portray success.

How does the medical community respond to these new revelations? Dr. Peter D. Vash,[9] Assistant Clinical Professor of Medicine at UCLA, says that overweight "is a complex frustrating enigma that disillusions both patients and physicians alike. Sometimes, I feel . . . the patient is treated like an abused child—nobody really cares about them until something tragic happens, or until somebody can exploit them. They should be treated only by those professionals who are best able to give support and care in a competent and compassionate manner."

On the weight-loss programs in specific, Dr. Vash says, "I believe that weight-loss programs and/or products should: First, do no harm; second, not be fraudulent; third, be responsible for providing some *definite and definable nutritional benefit to the consumer*; and fourth, be strictly held responsible and liable for the truthfulness of their advertisements, commercials, and claims" (emphasis added).

I would add one more criterion to Dr. Vash's standard: To be promoted as a weight-loss organization, I believe, they should be able to produce long-term weight loss.

Loss of lean body mass is of particular concern when weight is regained, because fat returns easily, but replacing protein is a slow process that requires careful calorie control to avoid adding more fat than ever.[10]

The following is a list of side effects related to rapid weight loss:

- obstruction—following stomach or intestinal surgery for weight loss.
- vomiting
- infections
- hemorrhage
- tooth decay
- hormonal changes
- metabolic abnormalities
- diarrhea
- malnutrition often resulting in hair loss and skin-tone decline
- progressive liver disease

- depression
- weakness
- discomfort
- electrolyte losses
- arthritis
- hernias
- leaks following surgery
- anemia
- rapid pulse
- abdominal pain
- overeating and weight regain, leading to weight cycling,
- death

When Things Go Wrong

Do the programs provide support, compassion—even when the dieter is not losing? Or is blame fixed on the dieter? What about negative health effects?

"Sherri" from Florida was interviewed by the congressional committee in search of the truth about her heartbreaking experience.

Sherri looked for a weight-loss program and chose one of the most famous—Nutri/System. She was concerned about her high blood pressure, and was assured by a counselor that her health was in competent hands—that she had "nothing to worry about." Sherri left it up to the program's counselor to tell her how much weight she ought to lose, and at what rate, and still stay healthy.

"I did lose weight, and very quickly at that," Sherri reports. "Almost ten pounds the first week." When no one at Nutri/System told her that rapid weight loss was dangerous, especially given her condition, she continued. Take note that none of their "professional" counselors warned her to take it easy and slowly. No one even mentioned potential health problems.

After some weeks in the program, Sherri found herself in excruciating pain, suddenly, in the middle of the night. Severe chest pains woke her, and her panicked husband called the paramedics. Fortunately, Sherri was not having a heart attack, as she feared, but a gall bladder attack. A few days later she had surgery.

When she went back to Nutri/System, she was told that her weight had caused the problem, *despite the fact that reports show gall bladder emergencies often follow rapid weight loss*, such as she had experienced. No follow-up counseling or emotional support was offered.

Sherri dropped out of Nutri/System. She was afraid, and had lost her confidence in the program. "I didn't trust them anymore," she said.[11]

Though she is only one example, Sherri represents countless others who are beginning to realize the failure of such commercial programs and are speaking out:

- Eighteen women have filed charges against Nutri/System after suffering gall bladder problems following rapid weight loss on the program. Nutri/System is fighting back with a national ad campaign stating that gall bladder disease is a result of obesity, not weight loss, even though none of the women had symptoms before the N/S program.[12] Nutri/System's president and CEO, A. Donald McCulloch, Jr., denied the allegations. "No scientific study," he said, "demonstrates that the N/S program increases the risk of gallstones."[13] Over 1500 calls have come into the offices of the attorneys handling the Nutri/System cases in Florida from former N/S clients and their lawyers.[14]

- In 1988, Nutri/System started a "Health and Fitness Information Bureau" that pumps out press releases to health and lifestyle editors of local newspapers. Their releases warn of the dangers of obesity as though it were the black plague. The "Bureau" also reports on the latest scientific studies by members of the National Health Sciences Advisory Board and National Health and Fitness Foundation, two official-sounding organizations that are actually funded by Nutri/System and packed with university professors on the company's payroll.[15]

- Diet Center's Jim Lijenquist, when challenged on advertising claims and tactics: "It's not the kind of advertising we like to do. We've been forced into a more flamboyant advertising practice in order to compete in this industry. If we were to advertise exactly what's necessary to lose weight and keep it off—commitment and hard work—no one would listen."[16]

- Some of the most effective marketing comes from Nutri/System, which A. Donald McCulloch, Jr., a former marketing executive with Pizza Hut, bought with some colleagues in 1986. It uses black and white "before and after" ads to show how customers have shed their fat. It also buys local radio time, then offers free Nutri/System diet programs to the station disk jockeys: (McCulloch put more than 1,000 disc jockeys around the country on the weight-loss regimen free of charge.[17]) The deejays chatter about the weight they lose and the tastiness of the pre-packaged Nutri/System foods that dieters must buy.[18]

- Most of the big commercial centers have changed their advertising and no longer promise rapid weight loss. In one of Jenny Craig's former ads the client lost close to four pounds a week—almost twice as much as what experts consider safe. In a more recent ad, the woman's weight loss is still emphasized, but the amount of time it took her to lose it isn't mentioned. Same ad, different message.[19]

- Former Nutri/System ads promise to help you drop two sizes in less than three weeks. Recent ads have shifted from the quick-loss guarantees. New ads have been introduced that tout the program's "scientifically established principles," with the slogan—"There's a right way to lose weight"—that is careful not to promise success.[20] Unfortunately there are no published studies that compare the effectiveness of various popular weight-loss programs.[21]

- Weight Watchers boasts three million lifetime members, clients who have lost weight and kept it off. But ask the company—or any of the commercial weight-loss programs—what its dropout rates are, or how many former clients have kept their slimmer figures for five years or longer, and you'll get an unsettling silence. No one has collected that kind of data.[22]

- What makes the diet business so lucrative is that there is no long-term cure for the truly overweight. Studies show that within five years most dieters are likely to gain back any weight they lose.[23] McCulloch's Nutri/System, as with all the leading commercial weight-loss programs, is creating a base of repeat customers,[24] and they know it.

- David Garner, a psychologist at Michigan State University who has long studied obesity and eating disorders, says, "The reality is that 95% of dieters in commercial programs fail."[25]
- The Diet Workshop promotes the use of vitamin and mineral support that are "intended to alleviate hunger and relieve physical stress caused by dieting, although there is no scientific evidence to back these claims."[26]
- Physicians Weight-Loss Centers say vitamin/mineral supplements are necessary for nutritional adequacy. Reliance on a nonfat protein supplement instead of food offers no weight loss or health advantages and makes the diet overly restrictive.[27]
- Diet Center recommends 1000 mg. of vitamin C daily. The megadose of C offers no health benefits and could carry risks for some individuals. Also required are "Diet Center Supplements" claimed to keep blood sugar levels stable and reduce stress. But there is little scientific basis for these claims.[28]
- Several experts not only question the substitution of supplements for food, but say that the use of the Diet Center Supplement has no scientific basis.[29]
- National diet programs haven't been adequately evaluated. For example, there are only two existing studies done on Diet Center and both were done by or financed by the program. One enrolled only 15 people for a mere eight-week period. With over 2,300 franchised centers in the U.S., Canada, The United Kingdom, Guam, Singapore, and Australia, one would assume a more thorough study would be possible.[30]
- Leaders are experts on the Weight Watchers Program at WW International; they're not nutritionists.[31]
- Even though an estimated 83% of the people enrolled in any diet program drop out[32], the revenues of a *single* Jenny Craig or Nutri/System outlet are an average of

$600,000 to $2 million a year.[33]

- Nutri/System, the fastest growing chain, processes 300,000 clients a week through approximately four hundred corporate-owned outlets and 1,400 franchises. In July 1989, it reported a 93% growth in annual sales over the previous year, to $764 million, with a net income of $50 million. In addition to the initial fee, a week's supply of Nutri/System's foods, snacks and Flavor Enhancers can cost as much as $75.[34]
- Nutri/System franchisee David Skulnik jokes, "I'm ecstatic, because my biggest problem is writing my seven-figure royalty check."[35]

Whom Can We Trust?

While we have singled out Nutri/System's attitude toward Sherri's health complications for the sake of example, keep in mind that their response reflects thinking across the whole diet industry: Health problems are not *their* problem.

Jenny Craig International, as represented by Ellen Destray, vice president, says, ". . . clients fill out a health questionnaire and participants who are basically healthy need not have their physician's approval." Approval is not the question, however. Anyone who is trying to alter or maintain weight should *consult regularly* with their physician, keeping in mind that health is every bit as important as weight loss.

Destray, however, reveals a lack of up-to-date knowledge on the essential need to involve individuals in healthy diet choices. In fact, some of her assumptions reveal an attitude that is demeaning to overweight people—that something is wrong with our ability to make wise choices. Consider her comments during the congressional investigations:

> Our menus serve three purposes. First, they take away the need to make decisions about what to eat, and clients at their halfway point are returned gradually to planning their own meals. Overweight clients have demonstrated their inability to make appropriate decisions. . . .[36]

Quite the opposite from the sympathetic, even teary Jenny Craig who appears in the TV commercials.

It is both unfair and dangerous to stereotype—to insist that overweight people "demonstrate an inability to make appropriate decisions" simply based on the fact we are larger than average. And a plan that's good for you is not necessarily good for me. On the very surface of the program—not to mention the mentality—to walk in the doors of Jenny Craig and other programs is to have your individuality ignored.

Time for a Change

Many of us have paid several hundred or even several thousand dollars to let someone else make our food decisions, retrain us in "proper" eating habits—only to experience the pain of regain. Before you repeat this cycle again, maybe it's time to rethink your approach to weight control, and to your *self.*

Even the weight-loss industry is being pushed to a new kind of honesty and self-examination. Diet Center, for instance, is now complaining that their "fair share" of the weight-loss market is declining because "we cannot compete in the increased volume of exaggerated advertising claims and promises being made by others."[37] How ironic.

Yes, once we believed the ads that promise "it's so easy, anyone can do it," and accepted blame for being part of the 95% who regain. But for some of us, that is changing: *We are not going back.*

While the clinics and commercial programs may be more of an emotional support than we find elsewhere, the health risks are too great, and the expense of failure too costly in money and emotional well-being. The centers and clinics do not deliver what they promise, and this is at their own admission.

At this point, the temptation is to ask, "If I can't do it by myself—if I can't do it with the 'weight-loss professionals,' then it's hopeless. Where do I go from here?"

One avenue—which I have traveled myself—is to seek help from the medical profession. Surely those who tell us the most about the health risks of being overweight must have some safe, helpful answers. Perhaps the news that we bring from the world of medicine will surprise you most of all.

Notes on Chapter Five

1. Lynn Minton, *Parade Magazine*, Nov. 4, 1990, p. 16.
2. *Journal on Obesity and Health Newsletter* Francis M. Berg, editor.
3. This information is taken from testimony presented at the hearing before the Subcommittee on Regulation, Business Opportunities, and Energy of the Committee on Small Business, House of Representatives, Washington, D.C., March 26, 1990. Hon. Ron Wyden, chairman.
4. Sources: *Fat Chance in a Thin World*, a *Nova* video; *Journal on Obesity and Health Newsletter*, Francis M. Berg, editor; *Health Letter*, Tufts University.
5. Transcript of the March 26, 1990 hearing, p. 1.
6. Repeated testimony and concern throughout the hearings by more than a few expert witnesses, Subcommittee hearings, "Deception and Fraud in the Diet Industry, Parts I and II."
7. It has been calculated that a person losing weight at Nutri/System, who wants to lose 99 pounds, would spend approximately $3000.00 on food products if they lost weight at a reasonable rate of 1 to 1½ pounds per week. "Deception and Fraud in the Diet Industry, Part II," May 7, 1990, p. 36.
8. "Deception and Fraud in the Diet Industry, Part II."
9. Peter Vash M.D., M.P.H., Assistant Clinical Professor of Medicine, UCLA, and President of the American Society of Bariatrics Physicians, in testimony before the Subcommittee hearing, "Deception and Fraud in the Diet Industry, Part II," May 7, 1990.
10. *International Obesity Newsletter,* editorial by Francis M. Berg, Sept. 1987.
11. From her testimony before the Subcommittee hearing on "Deception and Fraud in the Diet Industry, Part I," March 26, 1990.
12. "The Diet Business Takes it on the Chins," *Business Week,* April 16, 1990, p. 86.
13. Julie Johnson, "Bringing Sanity to the Diet Craze," *Time,* May 21, 1990, p. 74.
14. Bonnie Blodgett, "The Diet Biz," *Glamour,* Jan. 1991, p. 177.

15. Matthew Schifrin, "Living off the Fat of the Land," *Forbes,* Nov. 11, 1989, p. 194.
16. Patricia Long, "Thin Promises," *Vogue,* Oct. 1990, p. 400.
17. Schifrin, op. cit., p. 191.
18. "The Diet Business Takes it on the Chins," op. cit., p. 88.
19. Blodgett, op. cit., p. 136.
20. Ibid., p. 137.
21. Anne M. Fletcher, M.S., R.D., "Inside America's Hottest Diet Programs," *Prevention,* March 1990, p. 63.
22. Long, op. cit.
23. Schifrin, op. cit., p 186.
24. Ibid., p 196.
25. Long, op. cit.
26. Reider, Holland, Nelson and Mallozzi: "The Better Way," *Good Housekeeping,* Sept. 1990, p. 289.
27. Ibid.
28. Ibid.
29. Rebecca Hughes, "Inside America's Hottest Diet Programs," *Prevention,* April 1990, p. 72.
30. Ibid., p. 64.
31. Anne M. Fletcher, op. cit. p. 59.
32. "Are You Ready to Stay on a Diet?" *Glamour,* Jan. 1991, p. 176.
33. Blodgett, op. cit., p. 138.
34. Ibid., p. 174.
35. Schifrin, op. cit.
36. In testimony before the Subcommittee hearings, "Deception and Fraud in the Diet Industry, Part II," p. 8.
37. Allan N. Stewart, president and CEO, Diet Center, Inc., in his testimony before the Subcommittee hearings, "Deception and Fraud in the Diet Industry, Part II," p. 13.

◇ 6 ◇

Drastic Measures

Stepping from the shower, (carefully avoiding the reflection in the wall-sized mirror,) Jeanette heads for the closet. Why does dressing have to bring such discouragement? The blue dress is too tight. Also the brown skirt and cream silk blouse. The navy slacks cut in at her waist. . . . Dismally, she reaches for the same bulky dress she wore to work yesterday—and three days last week. She tried the rigid discipline of a popular weight-loss program but found herself feeling sick.

As she works the zipper on her dress, she thinks about the article she read in a women's magazine, promoting surgical fat removal, with exciting before-and-after photos. *Today,* she thinks miserably, *I'll call the doctor today. Because I can't stand myself anymore . . .*

How much have I regained this time? Bill asks himself. He has avoided the bathroom scale for four months. Now for the bad news. *This could ruin my morning.*

Unable to believe the reading, he steps off to check the 0 setting. It seems to be in the right position, so he steps back on—280 pounds. A sudden knot tightens in his throat. "This can't be!" He is 14 pounds over his pre-loss weight—even though he knows he eats *half* of what other men at work eat.

"What am I doing wrong?" he whispers to no one. After trying everything, and feeling like a failure, he now thinks, *It's time to do something drastic . . .*

Like millions of other Americans, Jeanette and Bill have decided that overweight life is not worth it. Anything seems better than this merry-go-round of weight cycling. They want to be thin, maybe even want it so badly they are willing to take additional, even dangerous risks.

Maybe you have now reached this point—you feel so discouraged, possibly desperate. Maybe a physician has leveled an ultimatum. So you look at your options—like Very Low Calorie Diets, and fat-removal techniques, which seem to be sanctioned and even widely acclaimed by the medical community.

Unfortunately, those in support of drastic methods often down-play the cautions. There are other drastic measures that are more private—physical starvation, which we call anorexia, and purging, known as bulimia. All of these methods can have serious consequences, which we will now explore.

Throwing Caution to the Wind

I sometimes shudder, remembering a conversation with Linda, a friend who was helping me after a Free to Be Thin class.

The conversation centered around another woman in the class who had a perfect figure, but insisted she had a weight problem. Linda said, "Joan told some of us that she was taking several boxes of laxatives each week and throwing up after dinner each night." Linda paused. "Neva, at first I was repulsed at the idea. Then I felt angry that I hadn't heard about this sooner. Not to help Joan, but to try it for myself . . . I still want to try it," she admitted, in tears.

Though I definitely discouraged Linda's impulse to try such destructive behaviors, I could empathize with the feelings that drive people to this point. And I have come to understand the reasons why an otherwise reasonable person will throw caution to the wind when it comes to weight loss.

First, I believe, the person who perceives himself or herself as unacceptably overweight can cross an emotional/spiritual line at some point in his or her struggle. What mattered in the beginning—serving God, serving others, learning to be content with life and live in peace—these things can be forgotten in the utter frustration of a battle against overweight.

The goal of living for Christ is replaced by a new, subtler

goal, which consumes time, energy, and life focus—that is, the goal to get thin.

Even worse, the goal of living for Christ and being a witness for Him can subtly change, so that we feel we must become thin *in order* to be accepted by Him or to be a credit to Him.

So the wonderful relationship with God that began through grace can become a matter of struggling to please Him again, without our even knowing a change in attitude has taken place.

Second, somehow we come to perceive being overweight, or even the danger of becoming overweight, as a health problem that needs immediate attention. Maybe, as I've said, a health-care professional has laid down the law: Lose weight *now*. Weight is your *whole* problem. Lose weight and *you will be healthy again*. No matter what, *just lose weight*.

Maybe you are in the midst of trying some drastic measure right now. Maybe you've been seriously considering one of the medically supervised fasting programs, or surgical intervention.

It's urgent, even vital, that you know what you are opening yourself up to, even if you agree to a drastic measure under a physician's care. *Knowing the facts could actually save you from untold pain—could even save your life.*

Very Low Calorie Diets (VLCD)

Many of us watched Oprah Winfrey on television and wondered, *How is she losing all that weight? Would her method work for me? Will she gain it back?* Some didn't question *if* she would, but *how soon.* Oprah went on a VLCD, and her initial success caused sales of such diet plans to skyrocket.

VLCD's are not new, they've been around for at least sixty years. Introduced in the U.S. in 1929, they resurfaced again between 1954 and 1959, when complete starvation was also introduced as part of the program. In 1962, Metrocal was introduced with its "join the Metrocal-for-lunch bunch" slogans. In 1966, supplements of egg albumin were used in VLCD's to reduce protein losses. At the same time, studies to determine the optimum amounts of protein and carbohydrates to produce the greatest weight loss were conducted.

In 1976 through 1978, however, the medical and public confidence in such diets was shaken by fifty-eight liquid-protein deaths. For a time, the progress of VLCD's suffered a tremendous setback. By 1980, they were revived, as modern formulas were developed and marketed by specialized clinics, pharmacies, and direct-marketing, and made their appearances in supermarkets. Today, it is estimated that between 12 and 15 million people have been on VLCD's in the past 10 years.[1]

VLCD's resurface in the dieting world because they work—at least at first. Many distributors, and even medical specialists, applaud their benefits. They are defined as: a semi-synthetic liquid preparation providing 300–600 calories per day as a total food replacement, taken for seven days or longer, or the liquid products in combination with natural foods to meet a daily calorie level of 800. Sometimes they include a vitamin supplementation regimen.[2]

While VLCD's do carry some risk, if you've reached a point of desperation the much-promoted benefits have great appeal. They are twofold: First, rapid weight loss. The very low-calorie diet is an effective means of fast, *short-term* weight loss.[3] Second, quick weight loss can motivate and encourage a person to adopt more positive lifestyle changes once normal eating is resumed.

The benefits, however, must be weighed against the hazards, and they are great.

VLCD's demand *careful supervision,* and they are *not for everyone.* They can be hazardous when not carefully used, as too often happens. Even researchers, retained by commercial VLCD companies, now warn: "The recent and zealous marketing . . . could lead to yet another round of complications and death."[4]

These risks are associated with irresponsible use in three areas:

1. medically unsupervised use
2. the use of VLCD's by persons not severely overweight
3. prescription of VLCD's by physicians not properly trained in their use.

While many will readily accept limited health benefits as a result of using VLCD's—such as lowered cholesterol and triglycerides, improved glucose tolerance and lowered plasma glucose levels with non-insulin-dependent *diabetes mellitus* patients, lowered blood pressure in hypertensive persons, and improved breathing in those with pulmonary problems—they also readily admit there are *more hazards than benefits.*

For the general consumer, body protein and potassium loss while on a VLCD are of major concern, and can be related to heart failure in VLCD users. Other side effects include: intolerance to cold, fatigue, light-headedness, nervousness, disorientation, euphoria, constipation or diarrhea, dry skin, anemia, and menstrual irregularities.

Most disappointing is the inability of VLCD's to produce *long-term* results. The quick return of lost weight is added to the list of real risks, not only because of the damaging physical effects, but the psychological damage. The magic of the VLCD is gone after the first use.[5] (Other side effects of VLCD's are listed in Appendix B.)

The medical community is already warning that VLCD's should be monitored carefully by a *team* of specialists. Yet, this is not being done for most individuals.

The resulting health tragedies, now coming to light, include: severe physical illnesses being caused by VLCD's that *never* existed before the diet; plummeting self-esteem and sense of personal failure, setting up many individuals for eating disorders. Researchers now believe that anorexia and bulimia *may actually be caused by severe-dieting practices.* Previously, these two deathly disorders were believed to be triggered by emotions, and therefore, the answer was to get psychological help. New evidence suggests that "the *event initiating* the development of anorexia and bulimia is almost invariably severe calorie restriction."[6]

Whether or not they are the cause or effect of low-calorie intake, we need to examine the further effects of anorexia and bulimia, and their impact on your health.

Anorexia and Bulimia

Most of us now know the definition of these two illnesses. But how many would *identify* more with the psychological definition—the sense of looking in a mirror *at any weight* and seeing a "fat person" despite the slenderness of the face and body looking back at you. You may have just lost fifty pounds, but looking at your reflection you see only the weight you have yet to lose. Even though you may have never tried binging/purging practices, or severe starvation, there are reasons why anyone who is a life-long weight-fighter needs to examine these phenomena, and know the psychological symptoms to watch out for.

Jeanette experiences one of these psychological symptoms when she looks through tears at the reading on the scale, declaring her desperation to be "thin" no matter what the cost. Throwing out caution about your health, and making desperate or secret lifestyle changes should sound a first warning note.

A second psychological symptom of an unhealthy attitude is to consciously or unconsciously relate thinness to self-worth, and to acceptance by others. It's true that overweight people experience many forms of rejection—but so do others who are outside the cultural standards. Getting your "acceptance" through weight loss is a shallow and often short-lived experience, as too many are finding out.

Third, you may find yourself being faithful and victorious on your diet, but preoccupied with food at the same time. You make sure your family gets perfectly prepared meals, while you munch away on your own little salad or piece of fruit, marveling all the while at your own "control." Many "faithful" dieters report experiencing an obsession with food and its preparation, all the while denying their own hunger and need. Living with this denial is unhealthy, because it will not last.

Fourth, for many there is the sense that life apart from thinness is not worth living. This may be so subtle that it can be easily missed. Ask yourself: Do I harbor a secret idea that life will be "heaven" when I reach my ideal weight? If you feel this way, it doesn't automatically mean that you will become anorexic or bulimic. But it is a signal that your mindset has become out-of-balance and needs corrective attention.

Likewise, it is crucial to be aware of the physical symptoms of severe dieting.

The long-term effects of any kind of severe food-intake restrictions, from the "drastic" fad-type diets to starvation practices, can be terrible indeed. These effects can include: loss of teeth and hair, and potential irreversible damage to sex-drive and child-bearing capability. There are more dangerous, hidden effects that can only be detected by your doctor or uncovered when disease strikes, such as loss of "lean" tissue, putting the heart and immune system at risk, and blood disorders that can also be triggered by starvation practices.

Anorexia or bulimia is not the first step to *anyone's* plan to lose weight. Rather, it is the culmination of a psychological process, and now, we understand, possibly even triggered by a physiological process. It also begins by attacking healthy thought processes. Whether short-term or long-term, it is a process of death.

If you are involved in starvation or purging practices—or if you have seriously contemplated either anorexia or bulimia, *get help immediately.* Don't go to someone untrained in this area, such as a pastor or friend. Go to a professional in the field. There is a list of organizations in the back of this book that can help you make a decision that could save your life. (See Appendix C.)

While anorexia or bulimia gives the dieter a feeling of total control, there are other dieters who would describe themselves as being unable to have control. If they can control their *eating,* but not their *weight,* they feel out of control. When they expend as much energy as possible on restrictive dieting, exhausting themselves emotionally and spiritually, and then finally give in anyway, they feel completely out of control.

It is this sense of being unable to control that tempts a person to turn over control to another. "I can't do it," we may say. "I want to but I can't." And so we may head for the doctor's office, once more asking for intervention, even surgical intervention.

Surgeries

For the last thirty-five years, surgery has been used for weight loss in some cases. During the '60s, intestinal bypass surgery was developed, and it was used extensively. During a thirty-year period, over 100,000 patients have submitted to *jejunoileal bypass,* myself included. Complications could be and were severe. The mortality rate was unacceptably high, and most patients were faced with a second surgery to reverse the first procedure.

While the intestinal bypass procedure promised an ideal solution through malabsorption of food, the successes of the '70s became the failures of the '80s.[7] I was one of those initial successes, then I became one of the failures.

My process started with Karen. I met her at a baby shower, and noticed her boldness as she asked each guest for their unwanted frosting flowers. She gathered the pink roses made of Crisco and powdered sugar, then popped them one by one into her mouth.

"How can you eat those things and still lose so much weight?" someone asked.

"Because of my surgery," she replied. "I eat anything and everything I want. It goes right through me—and I lose weight."

I watched for an opportunity and singled her out, asking how much weight she had lost, and securing her doctor's name. The very next morning I called the surgeon.

On January 9, 1972, my small intestine was surgically shortened from approximately nine feet, to only eighteen inches. The recovery was slow, and so was my weight loss. It was after two years of the severe side effects I disclosed earlier that I finally sought comfort and direction from God and His Word.

For the few years I enjoyed living at a lower weight, the ultimate damage to my health was a stiff price to pay. In 1983, I began to show unmistakable signs of malnutrition. My hair was falling out, my teeth crumbled unexpectedly, my periods were irregular, and I literally became sore to the touch everywhere on my body. Even on 850 to 1150 calories per day I was gaining weight. A year later, the bypass was reversed. I had yet to face a long, difficult recovery.

It began with nineteen days of hospitalization and misery, as my system learned to digest food all over again. My only real salvation was God's comfort. One particular day, as I sensed I was fighting for my life, I experienced His presence in a way that I cannot describe, nor perhaps should. And when it was over I knew God was fully *with me*—that He knew what was happening to me and He would never leave me or reject me. I had chosen life, even if it meant living and serving Him while overweight, and He would honor and bless that choice.

As my health returned, so did my weight. But to this day, I live with a sense of purpose and future because of having gone through those difficult experiences. Yet I'm not immune even now, even knowing what I know, from having to fight a sense of defeat and discouragement because of my weight.

But my experience, in God's hands, has been used many times in ministry to others. Not long ago, for instance, I met Lucinda. She came to a seminar I was teaching in which I began to share information contained in this book. After the seminar she asked me to pray for her, because she had a rare blood disorder and doctors had warned her of possible death within a few months unless she had an intestinal bypass reversed. Fortunately, there was good news later: After surgery Lucinda's blood returned to normal, she became healthy, and once again was able to care for her family. She also regained weight—but she was alive, perhaps more fully than ever before.

Then there was Paul. He'd already had his intestinal bypass reversed when he came to a retreat on "Being an Overcomer." I recognized the defeat in his voice as he told of feeling fat and ugly again, even though he was spared death and was experiencing renewed health. The love and patience of his wife, and the acceptance by Christian friends were incredibly important to his emotional recovery.

Patty also had intestinal bypass reversal surgery, and came to a Free to Be Thin class afterward. With love, patience, and the support of her group, she learned to make healthy food choices, exercise moderately, and maintain her weight and a positive attitude toward herself *in spite of* her size.

Since the early days of intestinal bypass, several more procedures have been developed and are being widely used. The *gastric bypass, stomach stapling,* and *vertical banded gastroplasty* are just a few. These procedures involve less of the small intestine and focus on reduction of stomach capacity. While many are enjoying the success of surgical weight loss, many others are experiencing painful and disappointing side effects, including some lethal complications such as: perforation of the upper or lower pouch; or, in the case of gastroplasties, perforation of the esophagus or upper pouch. Leaks that can occur within the first 24 hours after surgery have a fatality rate as high as 75%. Other complications can include vomiting and gastric outlet problems, hiatal hernia and gastro-intestinal reflux. Some will also experience wound complications, like blood clots and pulmonary problems.[8]

Some complications have no apparent relationship to the surgery itself, but to the rapid weight loss and its effects on the physical, mental, and emotional state of the individual. Vomiting, very similar to that of bulimic behavior, is reported in many cases. Slow eating, controlled drinking of liquids, and often grinding of food before eating is necessary to avoid this most unpleasant side effect.

While almost all of the early intestinal bypass surgeries have had to be reconnected, about 25% of the latest stomach surgeries need revision. And while there are even some reported health benefits to the weight reduction as a result of surgery, the extreme need for caution is evident. Long-term studies of surgically reduced patients are not encouraging. While it has been the method of choice for thousands, it has been the answer for very few.

In the book *Surgical Management of Morbid Obesity*, twenty-two authors make it clear there is yet no final answer to weight loss through surgery. Any one of us who have gone through this painful process only to lose our health and/or regain weight agree.

Where Is the Hope?

I have taken time to show all the negative effects of dieting, the diet industry, and the medical procedures involved in "helping people to get thin." With all this intervention—where are all those formerly fat people three years later? Five years later? Ten or twelve years later? Most of them are still struggling—perhaps sinking into wells of private pain and turmoil, experiencing a deep sense of failure.

I believe it is time to reexamine all of our thinking, from the inside out, about dieting, our physical appearance, and our worth as human beings *apart* from what the scale reads or the mirror says. Time to look at a way to overcome this "dieting dilemma" that has held us captive, taken too much of our time, energy, and money—and maybe even stolen our health and happiness.

For all the bad news I've felt obligated to give you—there is good news! I have found a way out . . .

Notes on Chapter Six

1. *Journal on Obesity and Health,* Francis M. Berg, editor, March 1990, vol. 4, no. 3, p. 22.
2. *Obesity and Health,* Feb. 1990, vol. 4, no. 2, p. 12.
3. Ibid., p. 18.
4. *Obesity and Health*, op. cit. p. 17.
5. "Timely Statement of the American Dietetic Association: Very Low Calorie Weight-loss Diets," *Journal of the American Dietetic Association,* July 1989, vol. 89, no. 7, p. 975.
6. *Obesity and Health,* op. cit. p. 21.
7. *Obesity and Health,* April 1988, vol. 2, no. 4, p. 1.
8. Ibid., p. 5.

◇ **7** ◇

Living in Truth

In examining the diet and weight-loss industry—from the outright frauds, to the medical procedures—one message comes through: Most of the time, no one achieves the thin healthy body in the long-run. But the previous chapters have been difficult for me to write, because I write in order to give *hope*. My great concern is that you'll be left with a sense of hopelessness, when that's not my goal at all. Sometimes, however, it's necessary to let go of false hopes in order to get to the basis for *true* hope.

This is the point that gives me great pleasure—because I have discovered the beginning place of hope. There is an answer to the dieting dilemma—a way of life that can lead you into peace with God and with yourself, and also into good physical, emotional, and spiritual health. It begins with a closer look at the "myths" that have shaped the way we overweight people view ourselves.

The "Meaning" of Overweight

"You are overweight." For many of us that is a statement of fact. But there is often an implication that goes along with that statement. We've all felt it—"Because you are overweight, you are a second-rate person." Most of us can recall one or two of our own painful experiences.

For me it was an unkind remark by an uncle who said, when I was a vulnerable teenager, "If you don't get some of that weight off, you'll never get a date." This said to me, "Because you're overweight, you are unlovely and unlovable."

For a man I know, named David, the message of rejection

came on the day his junior high school coach put him on the trampoline, which he loved, only to have the whole class observe the way his chest and belly bounced as he jumped. This said to him, "Because you're fat you are worth nothing more than ridicule."

Cruel and rejecting messages like these are sent our way daily. Why? Because our whole society is affected by *myths* about large people that need to be explored and exposed. In our society, being overweight feels like a prison sentence. Like Nebuchadnezzar, our character seems to have been placed on the scales—literally—and found wanting. *Overweight* carries with it more than just the definition of "too many pounds"—but character deficiencies as well. These are as unfair as they are untrue.

Have you ever stopped to ask: What *is* overweight? Who set the standards? What criteria were used to set those standards?

A quick answer would be: There are widely accepted charts, used by the medical community, to judge acceptable weights. These charts have been previously set by insurance companies based on a height/weight ratio, but in fact the origin of this ratio is unknown. It seems that at the beginning, perhaps as early as the 1930s, The Metropolitan Life Insurance Company published the first chart, using for the first time the term "ideal weight." Somehow this "ideal weight" became the standard. It was not based, however, on sound health reasoning or facts.

There are other "standards" too, widely accepted in our culture, that are not based on fact—rather they are based on theory, or on the personal preference of "experts." Unfortunately these standards are unquestioningly accepted by the medical community, the fashion and glamour industry, and the Christian community as well. These impossible "standards" have greatly contributed to the myths that have defined your "failure" and mine.

All our lives we have let other people dictate "standards" and pass judgments about our worth, based on our weight and not our real, inner selves. Unwittingly, we have either given others the right or assumed that they had the right to define our worth, based on their "standards" or prejudices.

How many women have listened to an insensitive husband call them a "fat slob" when they're actually only ten pounds over their weight at fifteen years of age? How many are like Sarah, who undresses in a dark closet because her thoughtless husband called her "thunder-thighs?" Maybe you can identify with Janet, whose doctor made a cruel remark about the size of her breasts when she discovered a suspicious lump.

Many men will sympathize with Ray, who went to a dermatologist because of a rash on his forearm. He was asked to weigh, even though only a topical ointment was needed, and the strength of the prescription had nothing to do with his weight. But the specialist thought it his job to ask Ray, "Have you ever tried to do something about that gut?"

Certainly more than a few of us who have been around Christian circles have had to sit perfectly still while some preacher departs from his sermon notes to go on a tangent about the excesses of food being "the only sin you wear to church for all to see." Any show of pain or embarrassment can only be interpreted as the "Holy Spirit's convicting power."

One formerly fat man told me of sitting through such an experience while the preacher digressed into a "by-the-way" segment during his sermon. My friend was an obese seventeen-year-old at the time, with his adult identity not securely in place. The preacher expounded on the life of Eli the priest, advancing his personal opinion that Eli came to an untimely end because he was so fat. My friend says, "I wished for instant death, or just to disappear. I know now that something in me did die—my worth as a human being, as a soon-to-be man before God. In that moment, this preacher whom I admired defined my whole worth—or lack of it—by my weight. I was fat, and *guilty.*" Probably no one thought this preacher was guilty of using scripture to abuse all the fat people listening to his sermon.

How long will we give other people the power to define our worth by our weight?

I think we'll continue to do so *as long as we continue to believe that they are right*—that there is something wrong with us as long as we remain larger than others think we ought to be. Yes, we will continue to give away our precious power of self-worth as long as we believe the lies that are deadly to our sense of personal value. And as we do so, we let others decide whether or not we will enjoy life and living.

It is time to end this ongoing tragedy.

It's the Lies That Will Kill You

We have already seen that many of the popular beliefs about overweight people and weight loss are not true at all. For example:

- Dieting will always result in long-term weight loss if the dieter has enough self-control and discipline.
- Dieting and self-control *are* the only answer.
- When we fail at one diet, it's our own fault, and we need to try again—and again and again . . .
- Dieting is good discipline, anything less is being undisciplined.
- One diet is as good as another.
- Fad diets don't hurt you.
- "Diet" or "light" products are effective and safe.
- Diet products are always the best choice.
- What nutrients you don't get in your food while dieting, you can easily and safely supplement with vitamin pills or shots.

The above statements may seem like common knowledge, but in reality they are myths. Not one of them is true. There are other widely accepted myths that have affected both our attitudes toward *ourselves* and toward *life*:

- The overweight person is always an overeater.
- Overweight people could all get thin if they wanted to badly enough.
- Overweight people are fat because they harbor deep emotional hurts that they refuse to deal with.
- Overweight people need their fat for security.
- Overweight people use their fat to be excused from normal activities and responsibilities and, generally, to hide from life.

- Overweight people are lazy, undisciplined, careless, and unhealthy.
- Overweight people cannot become physically fit, and they hate their bodies.
- All formerly fat people regain their weight because they go back to sloppy, fattening eating habits—like eating in secret.
- Overweight people do not have good and lasting relationships, and do not make good sex partners.
- Overweight people are bossy and loud.
- Overweight people have a character disorder and/or a weak will.
- Overweight people do not resist temptation, are not motivated, and are mostly out of control.
- Overweight people do not enjoy full fellowship with God.
- No matter what the risk, overweight people should always try to lose weight.

All of the above are really "myths," false beliefs about being overweight that many of us have commonly encountered. Across the board, most of us got the message—from friends, ads, from the fat guy in TV sitcoms who always took the pratfall—that being overweight makes you a second-rate person, or not a human being at all. We have received dehumanizing messages about ourselves and, at some level, we've believed them.

It is time to confront these destructive myths, find out the truth, and go on with our lives as people of worth. It is time to go beyond our shame and find that we really are possessors of all the dignity God intends for us.

Confronting the Myths

Confronting the myths is painful, but it is also freeing. Don't hesitate to look at them because of the pain you might fear—be bold for the sake of the freedom you seek.

Let's examine just a few of the popular beliefs:

- The overweight person *uses* fat to hide from hard work, physical intimacy, or to be excused from normal responsibility—while thin people are more likely to be hard-working, physically intimate, and responsible.

- The overweight person is *not depending on God* for help, because we all know that the fruit of the Spirit is self-control, that thinness, like cleanliness, is next to godliness.
- The overweight person *harbors deep emotional hurts* that he/she does not want to face—while the thin person is more emotionally healthy.
- The overweight person is bossy and loud (or timid and weak, or angry and aggressive). In short, he is *a caricature of a human being,* not an individual with personal feelings, likes, preferences, etc. The thin person, especially the "in-shape" thin person, is a "stronger individual."

Are any of these statements true? More importantly, how have they affected you? That is to ask, at what level do you believe them? And beyond that—have they limited you in living a healthy life physically, emotionally, or spiritually?

It is generally believed that the overweight person uses his fat in some way to his/her advantage. In a recent social conversation with a Christian counselor, I was asked, "Do you think you *need* your fat, Neva?" I was polite, and even quite calm when I answered, "I really don't think so, sir." Underneath I was disappointed that someone in a caring profession could be so uncaring. But my friend the psychologist is not the only one to use this approach. Books have been written claiming that overweight is being used by some women to avoid sexual intimacy. Using their fat, they "turn off men who would normally pay attention to them."

Sometimes the overweight person is perceived as *using* fat as an excuse to get out of work. They are accused of using excuses such as: "I might fall; I can't keep up; I can't bend over; I get tired. . . ."

The implication is that being fat has become *rewarding,* allowing them to get out of activities they find unpleasant (like sex, work, or responsibility). Therefore, the myth continues, that even though their size is unpleasant and may affect other parts of their life, the overweight person *chooses* to stay overweight for their own *gain.*

There is a judgment implied: The overweight person *manipulates* their life and the lives of others with fat. He or she would rather be miserable and unhappy than face life like the rest of humanity and get on with the hard tasks of living. They may also be psychologically or emotionally unbalanced, unwilling to grow up and face reality.

The overweight person is also often accused of not depending on God. One major well-known ministry actually kept a record of every employee's weight on their computer. Weigh-in's were required weekly, and job security rested in maintaining an "ideal" weight. Several of the staff members were known to live on fasting-level food plans, while many others sought surgical solutions so they would not lose their job. Overweight was considered a "problem area" that did "not bring glory and honor to God." It supposedly demonstrated that those not "in shape" were not submitting to normal discipline, or to dependence on God.

This conclusion is sadly judgmental: If you are overweight you cannot please God, or be a credit to His work or name.

While the above examples may present the extreme, there have been other abuses of large people that I have personally witnessed.

One such abuse took place at a women's meeting. The speaker for the day had "a word" and asked all those to stand who felt God was "dealing with them about their weight." When about one-third of the group stood, he proceeded to tell them that their "fault" was a lack of trust and faith in God's power to deliver them from food addictions. He continued with instructions that if they would go to bed a little hungry every night, God would honor their obedience with a weight loss and a return to "normalcy." Some, he declared, needed to go on a forty-day fast, using only fruit juice, to show God how serious they were about being "delivered from rebellion and a life of the flesh."

Woe to the women who could not endure for forty days.

In another instance, Sharon tells of going to her pastor and sharing with him her distress at being overweight. His advice? *Stop eating.* He also told her, "Whenever you are tempted to eat, think of your husband and his vulnerability to other women if you stay fat." And so even her husband's sins were her responsibility. What an unbearable load! And what terrible advice.

Overweight people have been accused of harboring deep emotional pain. This belief says that emotional health is *dependent* on being thin—or the reverse, that being thin is a prerequisite to emotional health. If the overweight person would just get some "inner healing," they would find the world a happier place and would get thin. The underlying idea is that if only the overweight person would find healing, *the weight would come off.* Therefore, if you cannot lose weight you must still need healing.

This conclusion is also a judgment: If you are overweight, you are sick or broken.

The overweight person is perceived as being "not for real." Surely a large woman cannot really like lacy underpinnings and lingerie! Somehow an overweight man cannot be a real man who prefers the slim, athletic company of trimmer men.

This train of thought follows the track that the overweight person has no feelings, that she or he is not a real person. Therefore, any jokes about fat people do not really hurt, nor do careless remarks (or inappropriate intrusions into the topic of dieting and weight loss as dinner conversation). Overweight people are subject to the prejudice of unthinking individuals who judge the large person less than human.

The Message of the Myths

By now, I believe you can see that behind the myths about overweight people there lies a harmful force: the damaging force of judgment. At some level, we know we are judged by others. And as long as we believe them, we will continue to feel second-class, dehumanized.

The sad truth, however, is that most of us have accepted these judgments: Secretly, privately, in our heart of hearts, we have judged ourselves. This is the most damaging judgment of all.

Christian psychologist William Backus, and others who

have pioneered cognitive therapy, tell us that one of the most crucial problems facing us—no matter what our circumstances—is living with a mind and soul that are poisoned by judgments against ourselves.[1] Judgments made both by others and ourselves.

Psychologist Chris Thurman, on the staff of Minirth-Meier, says it like this: "Most of our unhappiness and emotional struggles are caused by the lies we tell ourselves. And until we identify our lies and replace them with the truth, emotional well-being is impossible.[2]

"Simply put, lies are beliefs, attitudes, or expectations that don't fit reality." Dr. Thurman goes on: "And we don't have to go out looking for them. They come to us. We learn our lies from a variety of sources—our parents, our friends, the culture we live in, even the church we attend—and they make life emotionally miserable, even unbearable."

In order to break the hold of judgments against us, they must be replaced in our own minds with the truth.

To replace lies with the truth, we need not launch a major public campaign, nor hold a press conference. No, our freedom will come in a quieter way than that. The idea of changing whole societies' wrong beliefs about dieting and overweight people is too overwhelming. And even if we could change the way others think about large people, it would not be the same as changing the way *we* think about *ourselves*. Wrong beliefs must be replaced with the truth *in us*.

But first we must learn the truth, and then learn to face down the lies in order to walk in the healthy freedom that truth brings. Will you accept the challenge?

In his book, *Telling the Truth to Troubled People,* Dr. Backus says, "Jesus made the point that the question of truth is primary. It makes a great difference whether you know and believe the truth, or tell yourself clusters of untruths. 'If you continue in my word, you are truly my disciples, and you will know the truth, and the truth will make you free' (John 8:31, 32)."[3]

The first truth everyone of us needs to secure at the bedrock of our spirits is that God loves and talks to overweight people. The truth is that God says His disciples are those who continue in His Word, who know the truth. There is no reference whatever to a person's body size.

Dr. Backus goes on to say: "People are riveted to their problems and sicknesses by believing notions that are untrue; and they begin to experience freedom the very moment they believe and tell themselves the truth instead."

I would expand on Dr. Backus's idea by adding: Many people are riveted to their *weight problems* by believing notions *about body size and myths concerning dieting and overweight* that are untrue. I also believe that we can start to experience freedom the very moment we begin to believe we don't know the whole truth and begin our search for it.

In another best-selling book, *Telling Yourself the Truth,*[4] Dr. Backus says we must learn to argue with the destructive sentences we tell ourselves. We *can* tell ourselves the truth and use our situation as an opportunity to celebrate, enjoy and revel in the presence of the Lord Jesus Christ in our lives. Telling ourselves the truth means that we have to learn to replace the false ideas we have been telling ourselves with truthful ideas and concepts.

For you and me, that means replacing the myths about being overweight with the *truth.* We have to stop negative self-talk and start more positive and truthful self-talk. For the Christian, this is a vital part in the renewing of our minds, commended to us by the apostle Paul (see Romans 12:1, 2). Let's see how this relates to the myths and judgments we've believed about ourselves as overweight people.

Self-Talk

Self-talk, says Dr. Backus, means the words we tell ourselves in our thoughts. It is our interpretation of people, self, experiences, life in general, God, the future, the past, the present—it is, specifically, *all the words you say to yourself all of the time.*

What are the myths and half-truths you repeat to yourself? Which misbeliefs keep you unhappy and upset? First you must learn how to identify the misbeliefs in your life. Where do the lies and misbeliefs start? The answer to that is in your self-talk.[5]

We have looked at the myths about overweight people,

and most of us can probably point to others who made us feel worthless because of our size—but until we recognize judgments and negative feelings we are harboring toward *ourselves* we will never be free of the dieting dilemma. *Jesus Christ wants to set you free in the depths of your soul!*

Consider whether you have ever found yourself thinking the following condemning thoughts, or something similar:

> Why am I such an undisciplined slob?
>
> If I could only lose weight, I could respect myself.
>
> If God really loved me, he would prove it by helping me to lose weight.
>
> If I could overcome this [fear, anger, depression] I know I would lose weight. But I'm such an emotional basket-case, I can't get healthy enough to get control of my life . . . I'm hopeless.
>
> If I were only thinner, God would be proud of me and could use me to witness to others. Shaped like this, I am no good to anyone, especially God.
>
> I cannot buy new clothes until I am thinner. It serves me right for not being stricter with myself.
>
> Once I get thin, I am going to stay thin. Once I get this weight off, I will never put it back on! I would kill myself first.
>
> Once I get thin, I will begin a regular exercise program to help me stay that way. I can't exercise at this weight. What would people think of me walking down the street or riding a bike?

I believe that at a level even deeper than what the world says about us, we have learned to think very poorly about ourselves. In our own souls we reject *ourselves,* so it is only natural to look to others with the hope of finding a better opinion.

This fact came home to me so clearly one summer night when my husband and I were enjoying a time of relaxation in our hot tub. "Lee," I asked quietly, "am I too fat for you?"

"No," he answered, "you're too fat for *you.*"

He was right, I have had more trouble accepting my weight regain than he has.

Unfortunately, for most overweight people, there is little

affirmation to be found, and only more judgment to be heaped upon judgment.

Begin *Today*

Today is the day to begin replacing the myths and lies with a standard of truth that does not depend on judgment of our outward appearance. Even weight experts are beginning to voice their opinions in this matter.

In a book called *Obesity,* G. Terrence Wilson says that the basis for weight-loss programs are *not valid* if they assume: (1) that obesity is a simple disorder caused by excess calorie intake; (2) that the obese person is an overeater, more sensitive to food stimuli, and with a different style of eating than other persons; and (3) that training a man or woman to *behave* like a thin person will result in weight loss. What's more, he says, "There may be considerable benefit in telling them the facts—including the lack of evidence that obese persons eat more than others, the effects of dieting on metabolism, and that weight losses by any method are usually small and poorly maintained."[6]

But expert opinion is still worldly wisdom at best. The only place I know to get a correct, loving, unshakable view of myself is to go to God my Father, and to His eternal Word. In His Word I find that, though I sin, He wants me to plug into His source of *Life.* Though I lack, He has *provision.* Though I am empty, He is full and His life is *overflowing*!

Here are some examples of "self-talk" that may go on in your head regarding your relationship to life itself:

Thin people are more lovable . . . more worthy of love. I will deserve the love of other people only when I am thin, too.

Thin people can have fun . . . show up on a beach and feel like they belong . . . I will have fun *someday,* when I'm thin.

Thin people are more *confident* and *successful* . . . I hope I can get thin and "make it" someday.

Believing these and other such lies keeps us from embracing life. We have programmed ourselves to believe that if we are overweight, we somehow don't deserve life as much as a thin person. We are always waiting for life to *begin* because we have become convinced that life begins at *thin*.

We have robbed ourselves with our wrong beliefs about life and thinness. We have short-circuited our lives with destructive myths about the quality of life offered if we are larger than what we desire. It's time to stop. It's time to start living assured of our worth and acceptance in Christ Jesus.

Just as if Jesus were right beside you, right now, imagine Him saying to you, "Let me validate your worth as a human being. Your weight does not alter my love for you. I love you."

Choosing Life

In Deuteronomy 30, we find these words:

> This day I call heaven and earth as witnesses against you that I have set before you life and death, blessings and curses. Now choose life, so that you and your children may live and that you may love the LORD your God, listen to his voice, and hold fast to him. For the LORD is your life, and he will give you many years in the land he swore to give to your fathers, Abraham, Isaac and Jacob.[7]

"Choose life": When we stop accepting the lies that our worth decreases as our weight increases, we are choosing life. When we start living and loving others *now* instead of waiting until we reach our "goal weight," we are choosing life. When we open ourselves totally to God and His love for us, regardless of our *feelings* of worthlessness, we are choosing life. And when we let God be our life instead of an obsession with food or dieting, we are choosing life.

In the Christian community we talk about being pro-life. But do we include all of life? Best-selling authors James and Phyllis Alsdurf say it like this: "Being pro-life requires more than opposing abortion; it means taking a stance against all that stifles life and personhood. To be pro-life is to be *for* life."[8]

Let us adopt a *pro-life attitude* toward ourselves. Breathe deeply. . . . You are *alive;* you are choosing life with each of the following attitudes you make your own.

I am a valued, re-created being in God's eyes. First, let your choice for life bring you *new attitudes about yourself, your size, and your worth.* Let these new attitudes find expressions in your self-talk. Tell yourself:

I am living proof of the possibilities of being more like God in His attitudes of true righteousness and holiness, apart from my size. Begin to speak scriptures to yourself, renewing your soul with their life-giving truths:

"You were taught, with regard to your former way of life, to put off your old self, which is being corrupted by its deceitful desires; to be made new in the attitude of your minds; and to put on the new self, created to be like God in true righteousness and holiness" (Ephesians 4:22–24).

"Therefore, if anyone is in Christ, he is a new creation; the old has gone, the new has come!" (2 Corinthians 5:17).

Tell yourself: I don't have to wait to be thin to be new. *New* has already come, not of my efforts but because of Jesus!

I am fully accepted by God. God could not love you anymore than He does right now. Even if you could stay on a diet for the rest of your life and remain pencil-thin forever, it would not reconcile you to God! Jesus did what was required for that. I cannot earn loving acceptance:

"[For] God was reconciling the world to himself in Christ, not counting men's sins against them . . ." (2 Corinthians 5:19).

"You foolish Galatians! Who has bewitched you? Before your very eyes Jesus Christ was clearly portrayed as crucified. I would like to learn just one thing from you: Did you receive the Spirit by observing the law, or by believing what you heard?" (Galatians 3:1, 2).

Tell yourself: I cannot earn God's love through dieting, self-destructive patterns of weight-recycling, and negative thinking about myself. I can only accept this love through the blood of Jesus Christ and what He did for me. Our relationship is not dependent on my body size, or my opinion of my body size, but on His merit alone.

I can live in the Spirit, by the Spirit right now. God offers a life in the Spirit, apart from body size or self-efforts to conform to a cultural standard. He offers this Spirit life based only on His love and an awareness of my need. I didn't receive the Spirit by observing restrictive rules or dieting practices, but by believing His Word.

"Are you so foolish? After beginning with the Spirit, are you now trying to attain your goal by human effort?" (Galatians 3:3).

Tell yourself: It is not my goal to fit a culturally prescribed physical size, but to be like Jesus.

In Gilliland Glaphre's best-selling book, *When the Pieces Don't Fit,* I read these words, written as if from the very heart of God:

> My children get so mixed up. You think what you become depends on what you see in yourselves: your abilities . . . or lack of them; your opportunities . . . or lack of them; your successes or failures.
>
> Those things don't determine what happens in you and through you. It's what you allow Me to be *in* you that makes the difference.
>
> But you don't believe it. You believe more in what you *aren't* that in what *I AM.*[9]

I am righteous before God because of Jesus Christ. I am not worth any more thin than I am fat. Jesus died for me because I was a sinner—not because I did or did not deserve it, but because He loved me. Thin people are sinners in need of a Savior, too. Jesus died for me without restriction or reservation. My right standing is not contingent on my losing weight. I am a Christian because of what Jesus did on the cross, not because of what I do or don't do with regard to my weight.

"Not that I have already obtained all this, or have already been made perfect, but I press on to take hold of that for which Christ Jesus took hold of me" (Philippians 3:12).

Tell yourself: I don't press on to get thin, I press on to be more like Christ. I press on because there is waiting for me a prize that has nothing to do with my body size.

I have God's grace fully available to me. "My grace is sufficient for you, for my power is made perfect in weakness" (2 Corinthians 12:9).

Tell yourself: Even if I cannot find within myself the strength to be gracious to myself, I can rely on God's being gracious to me. In this time of being terribly vulnerable—as I learn new attitudes, and new ways of thinking and believing about myself—God's power is being made perfect in me, an imperfect person.

I am free in Christ to become all that He wants me to be—a victor! "To you, O LORD, I lift up my soul; in you I trust, O my God. Do not let me be put to shame, nor let my enemies triumph over me. No one whose hope is in you will ever be put to shame . . ." (Psalm 25:1–3).

Tell yourself these words of Amy Carmichael:

> Is it not a thought of exultation, that however crushed and crippled we may be, our Leader is marching to music all the time, marching to a victory sure as the eternal heavens? We follow a Conqueror. We "prisoners" of the Lord follow hard after Him as He goes forth to His Coronation. It is only our bodies that are bound. Our souls are free![10]

I can rest and be content with myself in God. "I have learned to be content whatever the circumstances. I know what it is to be in need, and I know what it is to have plenty. I have learned the secret of being content in any and every situation, whether well fed or hungry, whether living in plenty or in want" (Philippians 4:11, 12).

Tell yourself: I am not imperfect because I have an imperfect body. God is still doing a work in me and I am learning to be content while the work continues.

> He who loves as no one else can love,
> Who understands to the uttermost,
> Is not far away . . .
> He wants us to say,
> He can give it to us to say,
> "My Lord, My Love, I am content with Thee."[11]

My life is good because I am in God. "I am still confident of this: I will see the goodness of the LORD in the land of the living. Wait for the LORD; be strong and take heart and wait for the LORD" (Psalm 27:13, 14).

Tell yourself: The goodness of the Lord is readily available to me. I don't deserve it any more or any less than anyone else. It is available to me because He made it to be so. His goodness is dependent on His character, not my body size. Like Amy Carmichael I can also say, "As for God, His way is perfect—that is the substance of the words. And if His way be perfect, we need no explanation."

Life Unrestricted

So much of life is shaped by how we view it, whether we limit ourselves with lies or walk in the truth that leads to freedom. God's love is *unconditional*—and allows us to walk in the freedom of His acceptance.

Life is a choice—your choice and mine. We can choose to live today and stop waiting for tomorrow when life might be "better" (thinner). What a great tragedy it is to lose our lives because we are waiting to get into a smaller dress or pant size. We don't have to sing, "The sun will come out tomorrow. . . ." because the Son has come to our side *today*. He offers the blessing of living *now*!

In all we do, in all the disciplines we now embrace, we have a new "choose life" attitude. We choose foods because of their life-giving potential, not because we want to lose weight no matter what. We measure our caloric intake by our new "pro-life" stance toward ourselves. We choose to walk in obedience because we are worthy of a life of obedience. We choose to stop destroying ourselves, damaging our bodies and our emotions with restrictions and condemnation.

Tell yourself: *I choose life!*

Notes on Chapter Seven

1. Marie Chapian, Ph.D, and William Backus, Ph.D., *Telling Yourself the Truth,* (Bethany House Publishers, 1980).
2. Chris Thurman, *The Lies We Believe,* (Thomas Nelson Publishers, 1991).
3. William Backus, Ph.D., *Telling the Truth to Troubled People,* (Bethany House Publishers, 1985).
4. Chapian, Backus, op. cit.
5. Ibid.
6. Francis M. Berg, "Treatment: Opting for the Moderate Improves Results," *International Obesity Newsletter,* vol. 1, no. 8, Sept. 1987.
7. Deuteronomy 30:19–20.
8. James and Phyllis Alsdurf, *Battered Into Submission,* (InterVarsity Press).
9. Gilliland Glaphre, *When the Pieces Don't Fit: God Makes the Difference,* (Zondervan, 1982).
10. Amy Carmichael, *Rose From Brier,* (Christian Literature Crusade).
11. Ibid.

◇ 8 ◇

Choosing Life

If you think that I am advocating that all former "dieters" stop dieting, you are right. I am not saying, however, that we can all relax and eat whatever we want, whenever we want.

It is extremely important that we now learn to make food choices that reflect our attitude of choosing life—choosing foods and eating habits that are *life-giving* instead of *life-taking.*

I recently asked an Overeaters Victorious group leader who had gone through a weight regain, "What would you have to give up if you were to select everything you eat with a 'choose life' attitude?" The response: "The Snickers bar that I've been allowing myself to buy at the checkout counter, previews of the Sunday roast before serving, and maybe even most of the diet sodas I drink each day."

When questioned about the candy bars, she grew thoughtful. *"Why* do I buy them? Because I've been telling myself that I'm not losing weight anyway, so why not indulge? But now I see the answer to my own question. I see why not. Snickers bars are not good life choices, whether I lose weight or not."

Choosing life is not at all giving yourself license to eat whatever you want. It's a new attitude that says, "I will choose what is *best."*

"Diets are often a smorgasbord of prescribed regimens of uninviting foods such as cottage cheese and melba toast," says Debra Greenfield, a registered dietician and nutritionist in private practice who specializes in weight control. "A dieter eats these special foods until he or she either loses weight or loses faith."[1]

Most of us who have ever been on a restrictive diet can identify with Greenfield's statement. Though we chose to "diet," the severity of restriction was not a "choose life" kind of decision. If anything, normal life ceased to be, and food restriction became, no pun intended, a consuming daily grind.

Greenfield continues: "Ideally, weight comes off due to the reduced intake of calories. All the dieter has to do is stick with the program and maintain self-discipline. But this is not the normal way most people eat, and it leads to feelings of deprivation. The net result in many cases is an overconcern with food and body size, leading to compulsive eating behavior. *The best way to avoid compulsive overeating behavior is to reject dieting as a method of weight control*" (emphasis added).

No, we are not lining up to form a protest march, with placards reading, "Down With Dieting!" Remember: What we need to abandon is a *diet mentality,* not good, sound, healthful eating habits.

And so, it is time for many of us to stop dieting with unreal expectations and restrictions, and to start eating with our general good health as our *first* priority.

We need, first of all, to take the sting and stigma out of the word "diet" and return to its basic definition, according to Webster:

daily food allowance; way of life; regimen; what a person or animal usually eats and drinks; daily fare.

As we work at changing our mentality about the words *large, big,* even *fat,* let's also refuse to fear such an innocent word as *diet.* It is *because* we no longer accept the negative messages of being less-than-human because we weigh more than smaller-sized people that we are now free to restructure our destructive thought patterns as well as our eating habits, including both *dieting* and *overeating.* While we no longer carry or take the *blame,* we now find ourselves free to accept *personal responsibility* for healthful for-a-good-life food choices. Since balanced living sustains, protects, and encourages growth and new life, our food choices now bear out our commitment to life—regardless of the scale reading!

According to Jane Brody, prominent health writer, best-selling author, and syndicated columnist, "The time has finally come—the time to learn to live normally with food and to accept the body that results. While fitness is a desirable goal regardless of your weight, fashion-model thinness is not, unless you happen to be among the small percentage of people who are genetically programmed to sport a lean and hungry look. . . . If you are now eating 1800 to 2200 wholesome calories and exercising vigorously . . . then consider accepting your present weight as normal for you."[2]

"Our society wastes far too much time, money, and physical and emotional effort being obsessed with weight, and weight-loss diets. It is time to speak up for normalcy, and what is normal for me is not necessarily normal for you or the person on the bus next to you,"[3] says Brody.

Since many of us have been dieting for so long, to return to *normal* eating levels is unthinkable and frightening. To think of planning for 1600, 1800, or even 2000 calories each day is scary. We are convinced that if we have cut to 850 to lose weight, to go back to a normal, well-planned, balanced limit of twice that amount is certain to make us gain weight.

Dr. Wayne Callaway, author and weight expert, says, ". . . an initial weight gain might be experienced; it is simply a body reaction, not fat, and will soon go away if the caloric limit is kept up to recommended levels."[4]

What we see, then, is a new healthy attitude toward weight, best reflected by Jane Brody, who recently received the Distinguished Achievement Award from the National Association to Advance Fat Awareness (NAAFA). Following her award, she wrote, "We all have societally scorned yokes to bear, some more obvious than others. *We all should be taking the hand we are dealt, doing the best we can with it and getting on with life*" (emphasis added).

"Doing the best we can . . . getting on with life"—doesn't that sound wonderfully refreshing? To those two sentiments I would add: *Trust God for the rest.*

Unfortunately, too many disillusioned "dieters" think they should trust God *for it all,* and do nothing themselves. But trusting God does not exclude personal responsibility.

New Attitudes—New Choices

First we were programmed to think "weight loss." Then we slowly began to think in terms of "weight control." Now it is time to think of "weight management."

Realistically, if we choose life in our attitudes, we may also have to accept a weight gain while our metabolic systems heal. But this is not to say it is out of control—your weight is being *managed*. Because of previously chosen methods and programs that taught us to *diet*, we have *mismanaged* our bodies. While we may have lost weight, we have mismanaged our health. To manage our weight now, we may have to accept a predictable and perfectly normal weight gain. Thinness and health are no longer necessarily synonymous. Let's take a revised look at some more up-to-date tools of *weight management.*

Weight Charts[5]

If you have been around the weight-loss world awhile, you are acquainted with terms like *ideal* or *desirable* weight. More recently you may have heard the term *reasonable* weight.

As we mentioned before, the standard of *ideal weight* was set as early as the 1930s by the Metropolitan Life Insurance Company. In 1959, Met-Life revised their charts, and updated them again in 1983. As recently as April 1986, a set of Dietary Guidelines from the U.S. Department of Agriculture was published, offering a table of *desirable weight ranges,* listing ranges for women at only about three to four pounds lighter than men.

Today, the new USDA Dietary Guidelines of *acceptable weights* takes into consideration *gender* and *age,* much more than frame size. These weight ranges accommodate all frame sizes. Consider the chart on the following page. Where do you fit into the weight picture? This chart gives us an interesting view of the average weights of Americans.

New Goals

Choosing life, as part of our new weight management goal, means choosing goals that reflect *reality.* The American Die-

Acceptable Weights for Men and Women

Height*	Weight in pounds† 19 to 34 years	35 years and over
5'0"	97–128	108–138
5'1"	101–132	111–143
5'2"	104–137	115–148
5'3"	107–141	119–152
5'4"	111–146	122–157
5'5"	114–150	126–162
5'6"	118–155	130–167
5'7"	121–160	134–172
5'8"	125–164	138–178
5'9"	129–169	142–183
5'10"	132–174	146–188
5'11"	136–179	151–194
6'0"	140–184	155–199
6'1"	144–189	159–205
6'2"	148–195	164–210

*without shoes. †without clothes
Proposed wight standards USDA, USHHS.

tetic Association encourages us to set realistic weight-loss goals. Remember when we were on the old "pound-a-day" programs? *Not anymore.* The ADA proposes that a weight-loss goal of *not more than one-half to two-thirds of a pound per week* is reasonable. This rate will promote long-term weight loss of body fat, not just the loss of water weight, which is regained quickly.

New Calorie Limits

For those of us used to eating 850 to 1150 calories per day, the new information is quite shocking. In addition to Jane Brody's comments mentioned earlier in this chapter, the ADA recommends *10 calories per pound of your present weight.* Yes, multiply your current body weight by 10. For example, a 140-pound woman would set her realistic calorie limit at 1400; 160 pounds, 1600; 180 pounds, 1800 calories per day.

Dr. Callaway, the nutrition and weight expert already quoted, gives an even more personalized method by which

Average Weights of Americans
MEN

Height in inches	Age and weight in pounds					
	20–24	25–34	35–44	45–54	55–64	65–74
62	133	141	145	144	144	140
63	137	146	149	148	148	145
64	142	150	154	153	153	150
65	146	155	159	158	158	154
66	151	160	164	168	163	159
67	155	165	169	168	168	164
68	160	170	174	173	173	169
69	165	175	179	178	178	174
70	170	180	184	183	183	179
71	174	185	190	189	189	184
72	179	191	195	194	194	189
73	184	196	201	199	199	195
74	189	201	206	205	205	200

WOMEN

Height in inches	Age and weight in pounds					
	20–24	25–34	35–44	45–54	55–64	65–74
57	114	120	127	129	132	130
58	117	123	131	133	135	133
59	120	126	134	136	139	137
60	123	129	137	140	142	140
61	126	133	141	143	146	144
62	129	136	144	147	150	147
63	132	139	148	150	153	151
64	135	142	151	154	157	154
65	138	146	155	157	161	158
66	142	149	158	161	164	162
67	145	153	162	165	168	165
68	148	156	166	169	172	169

Note: These are the most recent national figures. Figures give calculated mean weights for each age.

Source: National Health Survey, USDHHS

to compute our new calorie limits, in his book *The Callaway Diet.*

Women:

1. Begin with a base of 655 calories.   655

2. Multiply your weight (in pounds) × 4.3   _____

3. Multiply your height (in inches) × 4.7   _____
4. Add together the totals
   from #1, #2, and #3.   _____
5. Multiply your age × 4.7   _____
6. Subtract #5 from #4   _____
   (Your normal resting metabolic rate)
7. Multiply result of #6 × 1.1   _____
8. Round off #7 to the nearest 100   _____
   (Your daily calories)

Men:

1. Begin with a base of 66 calories   _____ 66
2. Multiply your weight (in pounds) × 6.3   _____
3. Multiply your height (in inches) × 12.7   _____
4. Add together the totals
   from #1, #2, and #3   _____
5. Multiply your age by 6.8   _____
6. Subtract #5 from #4   _____
   (Your normal resting metabolic rate)
7. Multiply result of #6 × 1.1   _____
8. Round off #7 to nearest 100   _____
   (Your daily calories)

This requires some drastic changes in our thinking, doesn't it? You see, Dr. Callaway, who is former director of the Nutrition and Lipid Clinic at Mayo, tells us that we need to let our metabolism correct itself. That is to say, no matter how we have toyed with or dangerously altered our metabolism, Dr. Callaway's findings seems to reflect something we read in the Scriptures:

> I praise you because I am fearfully and wonderfully made; your works are wonderful, I know that full well. My frame was not hidden from you when I was made in the secret place (Psalm 139:14, 15).

For the believer, science's findings—that our bodies are created to heal—gives new breadth to these words also:

> Though I walk in the midst of trouble, you preserve my life. . . . The LORD will fulfill his purpose for me; your

love, O LORD, endures forever—do not abandon the works
of your hands (Psalm 138:7, 8).

For some of us, the correction of diet-induced obesity or
problems with metabolism may take a long time, and require
untold patience and mercy toward ourselves. But we must
remember, God has not forgotten or abandoned us. He will
help! He is the one who has told us to choose life. He holds
out life to each of us, but we must choose it.

Can you join me in new life-choosing habits? I hope so.

The American Dietetic Association tells us that the new,
higher-calorie limits serve four purposes:

1. to keep metabolic rate at a normal level;
2. to keep from losing lean body tissue along with fat;
3. to keep weight loss at a modest rate;
4. to keep from setting yourself up for failure and regain.

Once you have discovered how much good food you need
in order to *choose life,* the decision still to be made is: *which
foods to choose.*

New Food Choices for Life

Recommended Dietary Allowances (RDAs).

The reason we were designed to eat was to provide nourishment—energy to fuel our bodies for growth and health.
Therefore, it's important to know what levels of nourishment
we need to take in each day.

The National Research Council is that area of the government in charge of researching our nutritional needs. In their
latest release, the NRC defines what we commonly see on
food packages and vitamin jar labels—*RDA's.*

Recommended Dietary Allowances are intended to reflect
the best scientific judgment on nutrient allowances for the
maintenance of good health and to serve as the basis for eval-
uating the adequacy of diets of groups of people. They are
defined as: the levels of intake of essential nutrients that, on
the basis of scientific knowledge, are judged by the Good
Nutrition Board to be adequate to meet the known nutrient
needs of practically all healthy persons.[6]

What is the best way to eat, then, so as to take in the right daily allowances?

It is recommended that diets should be composed of a variety of foods that are derived from diverse food groups rather than by supplementation or fortification, and that losses of nutrients during the processing and preparation of food should be taken into consideration in planning diets.

Louis W. Sullivan, Secretary of Health and Human Services, calls the new dietary guidelines proposed by his department, "a dietary compass for consumers." There are seven guidelines to help us get our RDA's and achieve our healthy weights.

1. *Eat a variety of foods.*

A varied diet rather than a single food or supplement is needed to supply the forty-plus nutrients essential for good health.

2. *Maintain a healthy weight.*

A *healthy* weight is not determined only on the scale and weight charts and tables. It also determined by blood pressure, cholesterol counts, blood sugar readings and heart condition. If all of these factors are within normal ranges, weight may not be as important to your overall health as once thought. But before you go to your nearest medical lab to get tested, you need to know that your health-risk factor is also determined by how closely your hip measurement matches your waist measurement—your waist/hip ratio—or the distribution of fat in your abdomen, vs. on your hips and thighs.

Dr. Callaway offers a simple way of computing your waist/ hip ratio.

- Stand straight, in front of a full-length mirror. Using a tape measure, determine the distance around the smallest part of your waist. Check the mirror to be sure the tape is parallel to the floor.
- Still standing straight, in front of the mirror, measure the distance around the largest part of your buttocks. Check to be sure the tape is parallel to the floor.
- Divide your waist measurement by your hip measure-

ment. This is your waist/hip ratio.

You are looking for a ratio of .70–.75 for women, and .80–.90 for men. Women with above .80 are considered at risk, as are men who are above 1.0. Based on the newest acceptable weight charts, your general health and your waist/hip ratio, your doctor and a registered dietician can help you determine your healthy target weight range.

3. Choose a diet low in fat, saturated fat, and cholesterol.

Limit fat in your diet. Thirty percent or less of total calories should come from fat, and no more than 10 percent from saturated fat. For example, at 2,000 calories per day, the suggested upper limit for fat intake is 600 calories $(2,000 \times .30)$, Since there are nine calories per gram of fat, that comes to 67 grams of fat $(600 \div 9)$.

4. Choose a diet with plenty of vegetables, fruits, and grain products.

These foods provide much needed fiber, starch, vitamins and minerals.

5. Use sugars only in moderation.

Sugars and sugar-laden foods rate high in calories but low in nutrients, and should be eaten sparingly. Watch for other names of sugar that appear on food labels: glucose, fructose, maltose, lactose, hone, high-fructose corn syrup, molasses, and fruit concentrate.

6. Use salt and sodium only in moderation.

Americans eat more salt and sodium than they need. The National Academy of Sciences suggests that healthy Americans take in no more than 2,400 milligrams of sodium each day, or the equivalent of *one teaspoon* of salt.

7. If you drink alcoholic beverages, do so in moderation.

If our attitude is to choose life, there is also a moral consideration to drinking alcoholic beverages, in addition to a nutritional one. Earlier guides say one or two standard drinks daily appear to cause no harm in normal, healthy, nonpregnant adults. A newer definition of moderate intake says no more than one drink per day for women and two for men.[7]

Begin With Wise Planning

Motivated by our new "choose life" attitude, armed with the information on RDA's, and equipped with the dietary guidelines, we are ready to approach the market—to shop for health's sake, not for weight loss.

What does a *variety* of foods mean? What do I actually choose? How do I know I am getting the right *variety*? How do I know how much to buy?

That is where the ADA's exchange lists come in handy. They have it all figured out for us, daily allowances and all.

The ADA's six exchange lists help make your meal plan work. Foods are grouped together on a list because they are alike. Every food on the list has about the same amount of carbohydrates, protein, fat, and calories: In the amounts listed, all the choices in each list are equal. Any food on a list can be *exchanged* or traded for any other food on the same list. The six lists are *starch/bread*, *meat and meat substitutes*, *vegetables*, *fruit*, *milk*, and *fat*.

The exchange lists provide a great variety of food choices. Following your meal plan will control the distribution of calories, carbohydrates, proteins, and fats throughout the day, so that your food intake will be balanced.

As you read through the exchange lists, you will notice that one choice may be given in larger quantity than another choice from the same list. This is because foods vary in content. Each choice is measured or weighed individually so the amount of carbohydrates, protein, fat, and calories is the same in each choice.

Using your *target calorie limit* from the calculations you made earlier in this chapter, use the following basic menu to help you determine how many of each exchange you are to include in your meal plans each day. Then, using the exchange lists, plan your meals and menus and calculate the exchanges in your favorite recipes.

To help you get started, I have enlisted the help of Lisa Harris, a registered dietician and editor of *Current Diet Re-*

The Exchange List	Carbo. Grams	Protein Grams	Fat Grams	Calories
Starch/Bread	15	3	trace	80
Meat				
Lean	—	7	3	55
Med-fat	—	7	5	75
High-fat	—	7	8	100
Vegetable	5	2	—	25
Fruit	15	—	—	60
Milk				
Skim	12	8	trace	90
Low-fat	12	8	5	120
Whole	12	8	8	150
Fat	—	—	5	45

view. We have included in an appendix several menus from which you can choose, at your individual calorie level. (See Appendix D.) We have created fourteen breakfasts, lunches, and dinners. We have also anticipated various situations in which you might find special menus would be more helpful—a rushed breakfast, lunch on-the-run, and dinner out. Also included are suggestions for brown baggers.

Yes, it will take a little bit of work, but only a single morning, afternoon, or evening. Let me encourage you to create some of your own favorite menus, calculate the exchange values, and write them out on 3 × 5 cards. File them, or tape them inside your kitchen cabinet doors for easy reference. Use them in planning your meals and shopping. Once you have the exchange values calculated, it will be easy to keep your food choices balanced and healthy. Each six weeks (or twenty-five pound loss or gain), it will be important to do the calculations over again, adjust the calorie limits on your menu plans, and keep going.

You are now managing your weight! You have taken control of choosing life, health and wholeness for your body.

Use a copy of the following information to write in your exchange allowances of your own personal individual program. Update it every six weeks, as recommended, and keep it posted in a handy place for easy reference and motivation.

BASIC MENU

This basic menu plan has 1400 calories—about 55% from carbohydrates, 20 to 25% from protein, and less than 30% from fat. Each day, plan your meals by using the following servings of different foods:

- **Seven starch servings, preferably whole-grain**
  (1 serving = 1 ounce ready-to-eat cereal, 1 slice of bread, ½ cup cooked pasta, rice, potatoes, peas or corn.)

- **Five protein servings**
  (1 serving = 1 ounce cooked lean meat, poultry or fish, 1 egg, 1 ounce lowfat cheese, 2 tablespoons peanut butter if you omit 2 fat servings.)

- **Three milk servings**
  (1 serving = 1 cup skim milk or nonfat yogurt.

- **Three fruit servings**
  (Serving sizes vary. See the menu for some examples. In general, choose fresh fruit, unsweetened juice, or fruit that is canned or frozen without added sugar or syrup.)

- **Two (or more) vegetable servings**
  (1 serving = ½ cup cooked vegetables or 1 cup raw.)

- **Two fat servings**
  (1 serving = 1 teaspoon margarine, vegetable oil or mayonnaise; 1 tablespoon diet margarine or reduced-calorie mayonnaise, 1 tablespoon salad dressing or 2 tablespoons reduced-calorie salad dressing, 1 strip bacon.)

- **One dessert serving (now and then)**
  (1 serving = ½ cup lowfat or light frozen yogurt, ½ cup sherbet. One dessert serving adds 75 to 100 calories to the 1400-calorie Basic Menu.)

- **Unlimited bonus servings**
  (Because these foods have so few calories, use them as desired: sparkling water, coffee or tea, fat-free broth or bouillon, lemon or lime juice, vinegar, mustard, horseradish, dill pickles, Worcestershire or soy sauce, 1 tablespoon catsup or barbecue sauce, 1 teaspoon low-sugar spreadable fruit.)

If you need more than 1400 calories, use this guide:
1500 calories—add servings: 1 starch
1600 calories—add servings: 1 starch, 1 protein, 1 fat
1700 calories—add servings: 2 starch, 1 protein, 1 fat
1800 calories—add servings: 2 starch, 2 protein, 1 fat, 1 fruit
1900 calories—add servings: 2 starch, 2 protein, 2 fat, 1 fruit, 1
             vegetable
2000 calories—add servings: 2 starch, 2 protein, 3 fat, 2 fruit, 1
             vegetable

Food Choices*

Each day you need to eat a variety of foods. Each person's daily calorie and nutritional needs are different. A licensed nutrition counselor or registered dietition can help you work out how many choices from each food group are just right for you. By eating foods from each food group, you will meet your basic nutritional needs. For a healthy diet, each day you should have *at least* 4 choices from the starch/bread group; 5 meat or meat substitute choices; 2 vegetable choices; 2 fruit choices; 2 skim milk choices; and not more than 3 fat choices. These choices add up to about 1200 calories per day.

The foods listed in each group are just examples. Many others can be part of your daily meal plan.

STARCH/BREAD

Each of these equals one starch/bread choice (80 calories). You have _____ choices each day.

   ½ cup pasta or barley
   ⅓ cup rice or cooked dried beans and peas
   1 small potato (or ½ cup mashed)
   ½ cup starchy vegetables (corn, peas, or winter squash)
   1 slice bread or 1 roll
   ½ English muffin, bagel or hamburger/hot dog bun
   ½ cup cooked cereal
   ¾ cup dry cereal, unsweetened
   4–6 crackers
   3 cups popcorn, unbuttered, not cooked in oil

VEGETABLES

Each of these equals one vegetable choice (25 calories). You have _____ choices each day.

   ½ cup cooked vegetables
   1 cup raw vegetables
   ½ cup tomato/vegetable juice

MILK

Each of these equals one milk choice. The calories vary for each choice. You have _____ choices each day.

---

*Copyright © 1986 ADA. Used by permission.

1 cup skim milk (90 calories)
1 cup lowfat milk (120 calories)
8-ounce carton plain lowfat yogurt (120 calories)

MEAT AND MEAT SUBSTITUTES

You have _____ choices each day. Each of these equals one meat choice (75 calories).
   1 oz. cooked poultry, fish, or meat
   ¼ cup cottage cheese
   ¼ cup salmon or tuna, water packed
   1 tbsp peanut butter
   1 egg (limit 3 per week)
   1 oz. lowfat cheese, such as Mozzarella, ricotta

Each of these equals 2 meat choices (150 calories)
   1 small chicken leg or thigh
   ½ cup cottage cheese or tuna

Each of these equals 3 meat choices (225 calories)
   1 small pork chop
   1 small hamburger
   cooked meat, about the size of a deck of cards
   ½ of a whole chicken breast
   1 medium fish fillet

FRUIT

Each of these equals one fruit choice (60 calories). You have _____ choices each day.
   1 fresh medium fruit
   1 cup berries or melon
   ½ cup fruit canned in juice or without sugar
   ½ cup fruit juice
   ¼ cup dried fruit

FAT

Each of these equals one fat choice (45 calories). You have _____ choices each day.
   1 teaspoon margarine, oil, or mayonnaise
   2 teaspoons diet margarine or diet mayonnaise

1 tablespoon salad dressing
2 tablespoons reduced-calorie salad dressing

YOUR FOOD CHOICES
Calories Each Day: _____

Strategies for Preventing Habit Relapse and Diet Collapse

You have chosen the new "choose-life" plan for you. You have chosen to work with your weight in a management role, not to get thin, but to be healthy. Even though you have thought this through, made your commitment to life as prayerfully and carefully as you know how, you still will have days when your behavior will not match your intentions. You will feel like a failure—but you are not. It is not so important that you experience momentary setbacks. What matters is what you *do* with that setback.

This section is to help you on those days. Keep in mind, *relapse is not collapse.*

Change takes place in three stages. First, we make a commitment to change. No one can make you change, that desire has to come from within you. Second, we plan and take steps to make the change. Finally, and longest of the three stages of change, is the *maintenance* of the changed habits. It is during this final stage that your prevention strategies must be put into place.

To maintain your commitment to dietary change:

1. Keep a journal of your daily quiet time in the Scriptures.
2. Keep a daily diary of food intake. A list of menu titles or numbers is acceptable as an itemized list.
3. Set short-term goals that are achieved apart from the scale. Such as: having a quiet time and journaling five times this week; creating a new lunch menu with calculated exchange-values by next Tuesday.
4. Reward yourself for small successes—not weight loss but changes in behavior or attitude.
5. Line up a support system, including your family and friends, or a small group.

6. Purposely plan to eat one of your favorite foods within *limits of moderation* this week.
7. Shop smart by using a shopping list based on your planned menus.
8. To break a "plateau," either in your attitude or your weight, try taking a break from your routine for a day or two, maybe over one weekend. If you can't see yourself taking a break and getting back on your plan in a couple of days, simply go up to the next 100-calorie limit for a few days and give yourself some room to breathe.
9. Read good books on God's love, reminding yourself of His awareness of His children's needs.
10. Do not let your life center around your food plan and menu planning. Develop other interests.
11. Do something you have been putting off to do when you are thin. You are who you *are*, now. Getting thin is not what deserves your attention. Your *life* is.

If you feel that you need the affirmation of another person, perhaps a professional, to help you make the adjustments in your attitude toward losing weight and eating, ask your doctor to refer you to a registered dietitian in your area. This is an investment well worth making.

Many people claim to be "nutritionists," but registered dietitians have to study nutrition at the college level and pass an exam to be licensed. Would you go to a person for medical advice who claims to have a working knowledge of medicine, or would you prefer a trained, licensed doctor to treat your illnesses? The dieticians who have from time to time been available to me have treated me as a person of worth and dignity, in spite of my weight. They have helped me make food decisions based on my worth as a person and my health, with my weight being only a reference point, not the focus.

In addition to taking on a "choose-life" attitude concerning our eating habits, we can also begin to change our thinking about physical activity.

Perhaps you have been avoiding physical activity or delaying it until you feel *trimmer* and more *exercise-ready*. But contrary to popular belief, large people can become fit. The next chapter will help you put fun and life back into exercise.

Notes on Chapter Eight

1. Debra Greenfield, R.D., "Breaking the Dieting Mentality," *Environmental Nutrition Reprint.*
2. Jane Brody, "Personal Health," *New York Times,* March 18, 1987.
3. Jane Brody, "Jane Brody Accepts Award," *NAAFA Newsletter*, Aug. 1987.
4. C. Wayne Callaway, M.D. and Catherine Whitney, *The Callaway Diet,* (Bantam Books).
5. "History of Height-Weight Tables," *Journal of Obesity and Health,* vol. 11–12, 1990.
6. RDA's, Tenth edition, National Research Council, National Academy Press.
7. Special Report: *Diet and Nutrition Letter,* Tufts University, Jan. 1991.

"Just Do It!"

Who, me? *Sweat?* No thanks! That's my reaction to the mention of *exercise.* I get bored and I give up too easily. Maybe you're an "exerciser" already. For me, exercise is a discipline that troubles me more than any other.

I've often wished that a coach would knock on my door each morning with a cheery greeting and motivate me to get into my exercise clothes and inspire me to fitness. Of course, that has not happened.

No, if I am going to exercise, it will be because I make the decision to do so. The motivation, the inspiration to be fit will have to come from within me. I will have to come to a point where all excuses and laments are set aside and tell myself—in the words of a current Nike ad—*"Just do it."*

Why?

Exercise? Move? Yes—breathe deep and fast. Get that heart rate up. Sweat! But too many of us, who have been stuck in the "dieting dilemma" have asked: "Why? The weight doesn't come off. . . ."

For many dieters, exercise is seen only as something you do to lose weight. And when the weight loss halts, the exercise program can be abandoned as well. In this chapter, I want to give you the reasons, the very good reasons, why you and I can come to enjoy exercise.

In our new attitude of choosing life, we are now able to look at exercise from a new perspective: We exercise for *life!*

The benefits of exercise go far beyond those of weight loss. These benefits are essential to those of us who would now opt for the more life-giving approach of weight management.

Exercise benefits us three ways: physically, psychologically, and spiritually.

Physical Benefits

The benefits of exercise are more than physical fitness in the athletic sense. Exercise gives us general good health.

Physical activities, says a *Tufts University Newsletter* "Special Report," increase the heart rate—such activities as brisk walking, jogging, swimming, fast dancing, and biking.[1] This, in turn, can increase HDL-cholesterol (the "good," artery-friendly kind); increase bone mass somewhat and thereby possibly provide resistance to osteoporosis; and enhance overall cardiovascular fitness. These activities can also prevent or alleviate sluggish digestion, heartburn, gas, and constipation, since the muscles of the large intestine remain in better shape when the other muscles of the body are "worked."

Some exercises do not increase the heart rate significantly, such as weight-lifting, stretching, and the like, and do not directly bring about aerobic benefits. They do, however, improve the strength and flexibility of muscles, and enhance our capacity to work, play, and even to relax.

The Mayo Clinic *Nutrition Letter* recently reported on a study conducted at the Institute for Aerobic Research in Dallas, which showed a strong progressive relationship: People who are more fit stand less chance of dying from cardiovascular disease or cancer. This finding held true, even when researchers excluded other risk factors such as age, blood cholesterol level, blood pressure, smoking, and family history of coronary heart disease.

The good news from this report is that you don't have to become an athlete to reap the benefits of physical activity. You need only exercise *regularly,* and at *moderate intensity.* In this study, the greatest risk-reduction occurred between the "least fit" and the "mildly fit" groups.

And for those who aren't eager to do a lot of exercise, like me, that is good news.

Psychological Benefits

Exercise, the Dallas study reports, also cuts down on anxiety and stress, apparently by releasing opiate-like chemicals in the brain. This helps us understand how exercise helps fight depression and mental fatigue.

But in addition to the scientific evidence, you and I have probably experienced the sense of healthy self-control and order that a moderate, regular, exercise routine provides. These are important benefits we cannot overlook in a healthy lifestyle.

Spiritual Benefits

Since we are body, soul, *and* spirit, it is no wonder that exercise benefits us spiritually, simply because of the physical and psychological benefits. Our whole being is interrelated and each aspect is benefitted to some degree by improvement in any one of the other areas.

No—exercising does not make you a "better" Christian. All of us are in progress, all working toward better health physically, emotionally, and spiritually. Some of us have been at it longer than others, and some have made more progress, but progress doesn't have a thing to do with our *value* as Christians.

Yet I do believe that exercise brings a sense of well-being that God wants us to have, and it helps us to blow off stress and anxious thoughts, helping our souls to rest so that we can come into a truer relationship to God in spirit. Try it— you'll see.

The Fitness Fakes

As in dieting, the fitness boom has also provided a ready climate for the growth of fitness fanaticism and fakery. For example, the use of continuous passive motion tables (CMS) and the use of electronic muscle stimulators (EMS) have promised a lot and delivered little.

Developed in the 1940s as a therapeutic tool for polio victims, "passive exercise" proved useful for increasing flexibility by moving the joints. These techniques are still valuable for rehabilitation after orthopedic surgeries, such as a total joint replacement or ligament construction.

But for healthy people who want to get in shape, they offer little benefit. Passive exercise skirts the progressive ten-sing and exerting of muscles necessary for toning and growth.

Even though dealers of CMS tables claim that you can use them to lose inches, medical experts agree that this is impossible. Neither can CMS tables improve circulation—only active movement increases circulation. Nor are they effective in lowering blood-pressure or improving the efficiency of heart or lungs—aerobic exercise is still the simple key to cardiovascular conditioning.

Electronic muscle stimulators are another instance in which a legitimate therapeutic tool has been misapplied toward weight loss. In therapy, a weak electrical current that duplicates the nerve impulses that cause muscle contractions is delivered. These are helpful in reeducating muscles after periods of disuse, such as after a cast is removed. EMS, approved by the FDA for physical therapy only, is used to relax severe muscle spasms and increase the range of motion in injured limbs. Any claims that they can make you trimmer or more beautiful are false.[2]

Yes, I know there are those who would have you believe that all of life's ills can be corrected with a life of exercise classes. That is not true. Exercise is to be a part of a balanced life. Nothing more. Nothing less. But it is a part too easily overlooked or avoided. Let's not avoid it anymore.

Making the "Big" Move

You don't have to exercise to get *thin,* but you must exercise to be *fit.* Fitness is not size, but condition.

For large people who want to exercise, however, there are some special considerations and cautions.

A doctor's consultation and general physical exam is one of the wisest pre-exercise moves you can make. Tell your physician the kind of exercise you are going to incorporate into your daily routine, and ask for his advice. Remember, it is not permission you are seeking but *consultation:* How much? How often? For how many minutes at a time?

Those of us with larger tummies, and women with larger busts, should not perform the same physical routines that smaller, thinner people do. Do not expect to buy a high-impact videotape and be able to do it. A "choose-life" exercise program does not mean you should kill yourself. Use care; use wisdom.

For the large person, the unsuccessful dieter, and the discouraged weight "re-bounder," exercise is one way in which our self-esteem can be rescued. As coordination increases, awkwardness decreases; bulk gives way to grace. It *is* great to feel good about yourself.

There are so many options to consider when choosing the right exercise program for yourself. You are not limited to any one option; I encourage you to try many options. Variety staves off boredom and helps prevent repeating an injury or strain.

Exercise Machines

Of course, you could go right out and buy a treadmill, exercise bicycle, rowing machine, cross-country ski-machine, stair-climbing simulator, or a free weight mini-gym. You would not only be the proud owner of a new "fitness friend," but would be contributing to an exploding home exercise-machine market.

Home exercise machines do offer the advantage of convenience. But what do you do for cross-training, for variety? After investing several hundred, or even thousands of dollars, are you sure you would keep at it long enough to recover the cost and enjoy the benefit?

While all the machines can give you a good aerobic workout, so can walking, running, jumping rope, or a number of other activities. Remember, aerobic exercise conditions the body to take in and use oxygen more efficiently. It is essential for cardiovascular health[3], and for managing your healthy weight efforts. Home exercise machines might be helpful, but none of them are essential.

Worth investigating are the water aerobic programs offered by YMCA's and public pools. Swimming is not the only form of "hydro-aerobics" drawing people into the water these days. Deep-water running and other water workouts can provide aerobic benefits without putting stress on joints and muscles.

Exercise Videos

With the advent of the video cassette recorder (VCR), exercise videos have become very popular. Within the privacy of your own living room, you can have the benefit of a professional instructor, a simulated group for encouragement, and the convenience of your own schedule. Stormie Omartian's *First Step* is a wonderful Christian alternative, and a good place to begin.

After seeing *First Step*, I called Stormie. We had never met and I didn't know how she would respond to my suggestion—an exercise video for large people. Much to my surprise she was enthusiastic.

Very soon after, I found myself being fitted for costumes, working with Stormie to plan the movements, pick the music, and rehearse with her for the production. Our own video, *Fit for a King*, is now available through your Christian bookstore.

Fitness is not just for small people, but large people, as well. And large *Christian* men and women deserve their own program, designed just for them.

Walking

One of the easiest, cheapest, and most convenient exercise programs can be found right outside your front door.

Walking is an aerobic exercise that is pleasurable and almost injury free. It's easy to walk—indoors and out. Make sure you have good walking shoes and then follow these good suggestions:

1. *Make one-week contracts.* Set specific goals and write them down in a contract. Add a reward, if you like, and then sign it. Example: "I will walk five minutes, five days this week. My reward will be a new sweatshirt or bright pair of socks to make my walking more fun next week."
2. *Keep records of miles and minutes walked.* It's a great feeling to know that you have actually walked over 100 miles, or 200, or even 300.
3. *Watch your heart rate.* A good test for a training level is to be able to talk while you walk. If you cannot talk,

you have exceeded a safe level for you. Walking alone? Then recite your favorite "Tell Yourself" scriptures from Chapter Seven. Speak out the words to your favorite praise chorus; singing might be a little too much while you exercise. Keep increasing the intensity of your walking workout by how easily you can talk. You want to be slightly winded, but not unconscious!

4. *Exercise five or even six days each week.* Frequent walking will develop a habit. Three days each week should be your minimum target.

5. *Promise and give yourself rewards.* At the end of each week give yourself the contract reward. (One I love is to wear my sequined socks. I know it might seem crazy, but they're special to me—a wonderful reward!)

6. *Develop a 28-day routine.* By starting at five minutes each time the first week and adding five to eight minutes each week for four weeks, you will have worked yourself up to approximately 30 minutes five to six times each week.

7. *Begin and proceed at your own pace.* Remember the times you started an exercise program with such determination that you couldn't move without pain for the next week? Do not sabotage your plan with excessive effort. Give it time and commitment. This is a major lifestyle change of critical importance to you and your health. Take it easy.

8. *Cross-train, if desired.* Walking is excellent exercise, but it may not be your favorite. If you think you would enjoy another exercise after your initial 28-day work-up workout routine, alternate with other activities or exercise videos.

9. *Increase other physical activities.* Be consciously on the lookout for other times and places you could be active. Use the stairs; walk instead of driving; get up every hour and move around if your work keeps you sedentary.

10. *Don't let physical disabilities deter you from your fitness goals.* Consult your doctor and/or physical

therapist for extra advice, and find programs written just for you and your special needs.

11. *Consult your doctor.* If you have been inactive or are presently at medical risk, it is wise to get your doctor's input and advice. Let him/her be your partner in your fitness progress.

Walking has been and still is my favorite exercise of all.

Use the following chart to help you plan your new walking workout program.

While I love to walk, it is only one part of my whole fitness program. For variety, I have found it fun to use Stormie's exercise video *First Step* up to the aerobic section, turn off the VCR, and go for a short brisk walk. Upon returning, I simply fast-forward the video to the cool-down section. On alternate days I like to use *Fit for a King.* You could also use a treadmill instead of walking outside, or ride an exercise bike for the aerobic section.

When working with Stormie, I found it so encouraging when she would say, "Do anything, Neva . . . anything is *more.*" She was right!

Simple Exercise Equipment

No matter what exercise you choose, good *shoes* are the first piece of equipment in which you need to invest. There are many quality exercise or fitness shoes that come in all widths. Inquire at the larger department stores, and try on several types and styles before you buy. Don't be afraid to look at the ones with high tops for that little extra support so often needed around the ankle. Velcro straps help you put them on with ease. (Women can get plain styles or those with pastel trims, if you prefer. There are even good shoes with sparkling stones, for fun.)

A good *mat* is important when exercising on a hard floor. A good carpet remnant will work just fine, and can be purchased wide enough for comfort and security.

In our video, we used *a short closet dowel* for some of the stretching exercises. Be sure to sand it smooth and, for fun, paint it a bright color.

Basic Walking Program

WEEK	Warm-up Minutes (walk slowly)	Target Zone Minutes (walk briskly)	Cool Down Minutes (walk slowly)	Total Time in Minutes
1	5	5	5	15
2	5	7	5	17
3	5	9	5	19
4	5	11	5	21
5	5	13	5	23
6	5	15	5	25
7	5	18	5	28
8	5	20	5	30
9	5	23	5	33
10	5	26	5	36
11	5	28	5	38
12	5	30	5	40

Preferably exercise 5–6 days per week, not less than 3.

Your Target Zone

Your target heart rate, or best activity level, is 60 to 75% of your maximum heart rate. Higher may be too strenuous, lower provides little conditioning for your heart and lungs.

Age	Target Zone (beats/minute)	Age	Target Zone (beats/minute)
20	120–150	50	102–127
25	117–146	55	99–123
30	114–142	60	96–120
35	111–138	65	93–116
40	108–135	70	90–113
45	105–131		

Reprinted with permission from *Obesity and Health*. Copyright © 1990. Healthy Living Institute, 402 S. 14th St., Hettinger, ND 58639.

Exercise clothing

While expensive exercise outfits are fun and pretty, they are hardly essential; loose-fitting, comfortable clothes that have stretchability are. You might have a favorite pair of old knit slacks or shorts and a T-shirt: That will do. But if you dress it up a little you will feel better about yourself. Try to get a T-shirt with the name of your favorite major-league team on it. Go to the Big and Tall Men's shops and get a sweatshirt or T-shirt that will be roomy, and fun. Look for bright-colored solid T-shirts that are generous in size. Make the experience as pleasant as possible. Exercise *can* become a joy, instead of a chore.

"Just Do It"—But Don't Over-do It

Watch our for the "terrible too's": *too much, too fast, too hard, and too little preparation.*[4]

Attempting too much, with too little preparation, can cause injuries that wipe out the value of physical activity. When you find yourself taking up sports (which are supposed to be for fun) to get in shape, or if you believe that if a little training is good a lot is better, or if you try to "push through" pain to achieve significant gains in fitness or athletic ability, *watch out.* You are prone to the "terrible too's," or what is known as *overuse syndrome.*

When an injury is ignored or left untreated, overuse syndrome can lead to serious problems, including bursitis, stress fractures, and chronic tendinitis, which may require surgery. Prevention and early treatment are the best approaches.

Mild soreness, on the other hand, is often the natural consequence of using your muscles vigorously. A well-designed exercise program allows time for rest and recuperation. If you ignore decreased athletic performance (with or without pain), as well as chronic pain, and continue to exercise at the same level of intensity, you can hurt yourself.[5]

The physicians and physical therapists at the Mayo Clinic recommend these steps for preventing and treating overuse syndrome:

1. *Be realistic.* If you're past 35, or starting a program after years of inactivity, talk to your physician. Work with your doctor to set goals, intensity levels, and the rate of progress you hope to attain. Remember: Get in shape to play sports—don't use sports as a way to condition yourself.

2. *Start slowly.* Work gradually toward a twenty- to thirty-minute exercise period at least three times a

week. Warm up (to a light perspiration) before you begin the strenuous part of your exercise program, and cool down afterward. If you can carry on a conversation while exercising, you're probably working out at a safe level.

3. *Have fun.* Take up an activity you enjoy. Be sure that the demands of the activity complement your body size. Use variety to break monotony, provide for all-around exercise and lessen your risk of injury from repeated motions.

4. *Listen to your body.* The first sign of injury may be pain, swelling, tenderness or redness of the skin in the injured area. Pain is a signal. Sudden pain, or pain that lasts longer than a day, means you should stop or significantly scale down your activity. Never try to "push through" pain. Rest, not sustained or increased effort, is the key to recuperation.

   To preserve your level of fitness during recuperation, switch to an activity that uses different muscles but which enhances cardiovascular health. For example, if your knees bother you from running, try swimming for a while.

5. *Help the healing process.* Medications, ice, ultrasound, and the techniques of physical therapy can all supplement your body's natural healing process.

Eating and Exercise

For many, increasing energy expenditure through activity makes more sense than reducing caloric intake as an effective way to manage healthy weight. Increased activity promotes fitness and allows a more generous intake of food, which makes for easier attainment of the recommended daily allowance levels of nutrients.[6]

In other words, people who eat *fewer* calories may need *more* exercise to burn 3500 calories, because dieting slows their metabolism. With a more sluggish metabolic rate, a person must exercise more to burn accumulating calories. Put another way, a high-calorie diet generates a higher metabolic rate.[7]

You cannot separate the connection between eating and exercise, and exercise and eating. If you are exercising, you seriously need to consider the benefit of the higher calorie limits explained in the last chapter.

Do It—Today

It is time to make a commitment to *do it*—to take on physical activity beyond your present level. Make a commitment to do something *more.*

Just do it, and do it for *life*—your life.

Notes on Chapter Nine

1. *Diet and Nutrition Newsletter,* Tufts University, vol. 6, no. 12, Feb. 1989.
2. *Obesity and Health,* Francis M. Berg, editor, May 1990. *Nutrition Letter,* Mayo Clinic, 1989, vol. 2, no. 7.
3. Lisa J. Bain, "Exercise Machines," *Healthline,* Sept. 1986.
4. "Weekend Warrior, the Stress and Strains of Overuse Syndrome," Mayo Clinic *Nutrition Letter,* March 1990.
5. Ibid.
6. RDA's, tenth edition, National Research Council, National Academy Press.
7. "Calories In vs. Calories Out: How Much Is Needed," *Environmental Nutrition,* April 1989.

◊ **10** ◊

"Free to Be Me"

I have shared some very difficult concepts in this book, not to mention my own testimony and the pain that I've experienced. I've made every effort to give the best information and be as honest with you as possible. That's because I want you to know that I'm not ahead of, or above you in any way—I am *with you* in the struggle.

I am not disowning the *Free to Be Thin* teaching and principles upon which the ministry of Overeaters Victorious was built. But I now know there is more—much more to overweight than the "need for self-control."

Some who have read this far may be experiencing disappointment: That will be the case if you are still locked into the goal of becoming forever thin. You may be asking, "Where do I go from here?"

In Chapter Two, you explored a personal inventory of your experiences with weight loss, feelings about yourself and your lack of "success." But that was before you read the information in this book. If I were to ask you the questions again—have your answers changed?

How do you feel about yourself as an overweight person now?

Do you still dislike yourself?

Do you feel the shame lifting?

How many of the fraudulent products or programs have you tried? How many have your friends tried? Have you ever been approached by a close friend or family member about becoming involved in a multi-level-marketing weight-loss plan?

How much weight have you lost and regained? Are you

still willing to go on losing and gaining, with no end in sight for the destructive weight-cycling pattern in your life?

What do you now believe about God—does He love you no matter how much you weigh?

How many "myths" have you believed about yourself, and which truths have you decided to believe instead?

The Path From Here

Here are eight important things you need to know in order to proceed from a base of *inner change* to this point:

1. God loves you and wants to have a close relationship with you.

"For God so loved the world that he gave his one and only Son, that whoever believes in him shall not perish but have eternal life. For God did not send his Son into the world to condemn the world, but to save the world through him" (John 3:16, 17).

"The LORD appeared to us in the past, saying: 'I have loved you with an everlasting love; I have drawn you with loving-kindness. I will build you up again and you will be rebuilt. . . . Again you will take up your tambourines and go out to dance with the joyful' " (Jeremiah 31:3, 4).

"How great is the love the Father has lavished on us, that we should be called children of God! And that is what we are!" (1 John 3:1).

God's Word is true and cannot be changed. Even when we aren't happy with the way we look, He loves us. Even when we are unhappy with Him because of the way we look, He loves us. He wants us to come to Him, accept Him into our lives, and live in fellowship with Him.

2. The way you look is not as important as who you are.

"Dear friends, now we are children of God . . ."(1 John 3:2).

"The Spirit himself testifies with our spirit that we are God's children. Now if we are children, then we are heirs—heirs of God and co-heirs with Christ, if indeed we share in his sufferings in order that we may also share in his glory" (Romans 8:16, 17).

"For you are a people holy to the LORD your God. Out of all the peoples on the face of the earth, the LORD has chosen you to be his treasured possession" (Deuteronomy 14:2).

3. Your body weight may not be your fault.

It is important that we take responsibility for our behavior, but do not accept blame for being less than what society defines as perfect.

"Blessed are they whose ways are blameless, who walk according to the law of the LORD. Blessed are they who keep his statues and seek him with all their heart. They do nothing wrong; they walk in his ways. You have laid down precepts that are to be fully obeyed. Oh, that my ways were steadfast in obeying your decrees! Then I would not be put to shame when I consider all your commands. I will praise you with an upright heart as I learn your righteous laws" (Psalm 119:1–7).

4. Even if it is impossible to change your body—it is possible to change how you feel about your body—to be at peace with your own miraculous physical being.

"For you created my inmost being; you knit me together in my mother's womb. I praise you because I am fearfully and wonderfully made; your works are wonderful, I know that full well. My frame was not hidden from you when I was made in the secret place. When I was woven together in the depths of the earth, your eyes saw my unformed body. All the days ordained for me were written in your book before one of them came to be" (Psalm 139:13–16).

5. Negative body image is based more on how we think others perceive us than the reality of how we look.

"We do not dare to classify or compare ourselves with some who commend themselves. When they measure themselves by themselves and compare themselves with themselves, they are not wise" (2 Corinthians 10:12).

"But the LORD said to Samuel, 'Do not consider his appearance or his height, for I have rejected him. The LORD does not look at the things man looks at. Man looks at the outward appearance, but the LORD looks at the heart' " (1 Samuel 16:7).

6. *There is no such thing as a "perfect" body. Even if there were, it would never be a justified measure of worth.*

"[Jesus] had no beauty or majesty to attract us to him, nothing in his appearance that we should desire him" (Isaiah 53:2).

"Each one should test his own actions. Then he can take pride in himself, without comparing himself to somebody else" (Galatians 6:4).

7. *Almost everyone experiences negative feelings based on negative body-image ideas at one time or another.*

"No temptation has seized you except what is common to man" (1 Corinthians 10:13).

"Do not conform any longer to the pattern of this world, but be transformed by the renewing of your mind. Then you will be able to test and approve what God's will is—his good, pleasing and perfect will" (Romans 12:2).

8. *We don't have to live in extremes—we can live a balanced life.*

"So I say, live by the Spirit, and you will not gratify the desires of the sinful nature" (Galatians 5:16).

"But the fruit of the Spirit is love, joy, peace, patience, kindness, goodness, faithfulness, gentleness and self-control. Against such things there is no law" (Galatians 5:22, 23).

"Be very careful, then, how you live—not as unwise but as wise . . ." (Ephesians 5:15).

"Therefore, I urge you, brothers, in view of God's mercy, to offer your bodies as living sacrifices, holy and pleasing to God—this is your spiritual act of worship" (Romans 12:1).

Ideal vs. Real

We have been promised, and we have accepted the myth, that our quality of life depends on being skinny, blonde, and rich.

Ellyn Satter, dietician, author, and specialist in treating eating disorders, says: "The Cinderella myth has led many women to waste their lives waiting to become thin."[1]

Likewise, Frances Berg writes:

> All seem caught up in the current obsession with weight and body image—the fashion industry, television, the print media, the medical community, health professionals, schools, family, friends, and peers. All seem to be promoting or striving for the idealized body.[2]

But reality is found in the real people who live right around us. We are surrounded by people who are not skinny, blonde, and rich, who are living at a high level of life-quality. Those of us who have accepted Christ have been given a quality of life that does not depend on the *external*—but the *eternal.*

Isn't it time for a change? I think so.

Erma Bombeck reminds us: "At some point in our lives we have to come to terms with the way we look. Eleanor Roosevelt did not have the body of a nymph who graces the pages of a *Victoria's Secret* catalog. What she did have was one of the finest minds of any century.

"The symbol of our country, the Statue of Liberty, has a 420-inch waist, and she's breathtaking. Peter Paul Rubens' wife was termed 'ample,' but she was beautiful enough to appear in nineteen of his famed canvases."

What has made the difference in our current age?

Since the first decade of the twentieth century, the idealized American man and woman have become tubular, lean and slender—a figure that almost no one has. This increasingly "thin ideal" has created a self-image problem for the vast majority of women in this the last decade of this century[3] and, increasingly, for men too.

Experts may disagree on the causes of this negative body image, but they agree that the effects are obvious. They are also destructive.

Will we ever be strong enough to withstand the perceived societal pressures and prejudices to be perfect and appreciate just being ourselves? Is there a way to redefine the perfect body?

Perhaps Lynne Cox, five feet six inches tall, and 180 pounds, gives us a clue. A long-distance, champion swimmer, Cox has made her body work for her. With a smile she says, "My body is perfect for me. It just seems to work very efficiently."

Or, maybe we should listen to Yasser Seirawan, champion chess player. At 175 pounds and a hair under six feet fall, he regularly plays tennis, basketball, and kick-boxes with his girlfriend. Realizing that intense periods of concentration drain a person even more than physical exertion, he says, "To be in top chess form, you must be in good shape. When I feel physically well, I play good chess."

We must realize that the body that is perfect is the one that does the job. Amanda McKerrow, five-foot-four, 95-pound ballerina knows that. So does 235-pound mass of muscle, Alonzo Highsmith, the football full-back. Five foot four inch, muscular Pat Valenzuela has a perfect 112-pound body, for a jockey; as does five foot nine inch, 175-pound Metropolitan Opera singer Barbara Conrad.[4]

Our bodies are wonderful, most working almost perfectly. Maybe they don't need to be changed, perhaps it is our image of them that needs improving.

Free to Be Thin?

If I could change *Free to Be Thin* . . .

That is a thought that I have contemplated for several years. I know if it were written today it would be a bit different. The biblical principles are still the same, and they have sustained me throughout the years since. I live by them to this day—they are life to me.

But I would now enlarge upon those wonderful principles (listed in Chapter One). I would add to them:

1. Address the wisdom of higher calorie limits. Base the search for God's direction concerning specific limits on Psalm 139:14: "I praise you because I am fearfully and wonderfully made; your works are wonderful, I know that full well."

2. Emphasize exercise more and sooner. I would recommend moderate physical activity, planned with a per-

son's personal preference and interest in mind.

3. Take the word *forever* off the cover of the book, and redefine thin as a *healthy weight* instead of *ideal* or *desired weight.*
4. Place more emphasis on the importance of changed attitudes and behaviors than goal weight.

In altering the *Overeaters Victorious* program I now:

1. Train leaders to place more emphasis on spiritual quality of life, instead of on the physical.
2. Stress even more the importance of daily quiet time, accountability, personal responsibility for behavior, and obedience to God's Word.
3. Have a new philosophy of ministry:

    We recognize that dieting is a matter of food, but that losing weight is not that simple. We choose to learn to eat wisely and to exercise in an attitude of obedience and stewardship to God, empowered by the Holy Spirit. Being motivated by our sincere desire to please God and live in fellowship with Him, in trust, we leave the results to Him.

    In other words—doing our best, and trusting God for the rest.
4. Take as our ministry goal the words of Susan Wooley, Ph.D., University of Cincinnati College of Medicine:

    . . . to help [overweight people] come to some kind of lasting and permanent resolution of the weight issue. To find a weight that they can accept, that they can live with and get off this bandwagon once and for all. And to try to return to them some sense of dignity, self-respect, and control.

5. Encourage those who come to our ministry to stop spending their lives and energies waiting to do the important things they want to do until they are thin. And, help them find their areas of giftedness and rightful place in the body of Christ.
6. Pattern our meeting times after Romans 15:1–7: Bear with the weak, build up one another, learn from and learn to be a scriptural example, learn to endure, be

encouraged by God's Word, hang on to hope, and accept one another.

7. Make OV meetings a place where those who are suffering from the pain of regain would feel safe and restored.

What This Can Mean to You

Having presented this material in a seminar setting several times, I have had the wonderful experience of hearing the feedback concerning the impact this information has had on those in attendance. I hope their comments will reflect your own new heart attitudes:

"I've lived with so much guilt and condemnation that I was believing the lie that God had given up on me. I couldn't understand how He could still love me and be with me while I'm not where I should be. I now have light where before I had darkness."

"As an Overeaters Victorious leader who has gained back some weight, I really am ministered to by this material. I have felt like a failure—to the program, to the members of my group, to myself, and to God. Now I have hope."

"This has really healed a lot of hurt for me. I have searched for hidden sin, and knowing that weight regain is more a sign of a physiological problem than a spiritual one is totally releasing for me. Now I can look for a solution in the right place."

"This has helped me to know that I can now accept myself like I am and know God loves me, and I am no less a person because of the big numbers on the scale."

"My life has always been on the back burner waiting until I could lose weight. Today I have had 100 pounds lifted from my shoulders. It is wonderful!"

"Today, for the first time in my life, I actually feel better about *me*. I am finally free from my fat!"

"It's so wonderful to feel really free—free to be all God wants me to be."

"I am overwhelmed. I have really let the scales declare my victory instead of the Cross and have relied on what they have said about me instead of what Jesus says about me."

"I came with doubts, but leave with a hope and a future. . . ."

Into a New Light

Recently, I came across these words, which spoke to me deeply with almost a devotional quality:

> The early morning fog lay in the canyon, completely hiding from our view the mountain that rises just beyond [the nearby town]. When I looked out the window, it seemed like there were no mountains. The fog made it seem very simple. But when the fog lifted, I could see the peaks and the valleys, and the complexity of the mountain was revealed.
>
> And so it is with the study of obesity. We begin with what seems a simple problem, then as we draw the fog away, we find a great complexity.[5]

Yes, the fog is now lifting and it does reveal more complexities than we considered before. For you and me this means freedom from simplistic and unworkable "answers" that are not answers at all. With the lifting of the fog comes the release from shame and guilt carried by far too many of us—carried too long, and needlessly.

With the lifting of the fog comes hope. Hope burns brightly in me as never before. And—the greatest thing of all—it is a hope that cannot be put out by the scale. No matter what, I *can* trust God. And so can you.

These final words come from the beloved devotional classic, *Streams in the Desert*:

> If God would prove that He can give songs in the night, He must first make it night.

I have experienced the night—I have also learned the song.

I have learned to overcome the dieting dilemma. I am finally free—*free to be me*.

You can be free, too.

Notes on Chapter Ten

1. *Obesity and Health,* Francis M. Berg, editor, March 1989.
2. Francis M. Berg, "Obsessed With the Idealized Body," *Obesity and Health Newsletter,* March 1989.
3. Beatrice Robinson, Ph.D., "Fashions in the Female Figure," the *Melpomene Report,* (Mpls, Minn.: Melpomene Institute), Feb. 1985.
4. "The Perfect Body," *Special Report on Health,* Nov. 1989-Jan. 1990.
5. Dr. Campfield of Hoffman-LaRoche, New Jersey, addressing the North American Association for the Study of Obesity, meeting in Banff, Alberta, Canada, August 1988.

◇ Appendix A ◇

Weight-Loss Fraud and Quackery: Guidelines for Identification.*

Fraudulent weight-loss products and programs often rely on unscrupulous but persuasive combinations of message, program, ingredients, mystique and method of availability. A weight-loss product or program may be fraudulent if it does one or more of the following:

Message

- Claims or implies a large, fast weight loss—often promised as easy, effortless, guaranteed, or permanent. (Recommended loss for most people is no more than two pounds per week.)
- Implies weight can be lost without restricting calories or exercising, and discounts the benefits of exercise.
- Uses typical quackery terms such as: miraculous, breakthrough, exclusive, secret, unique, ancient, accidental discovery, doctor developed.
- Claims to get rid of "cellulite." (Cellulite does not exist, and reference to it is a red flag warning of fraud or misinformation.)
- Relies heavily on undocumented case histories, before and after photos, and testimonials by "satisfied customers" (who are often paid for testimony, which is written by the advertiser.)
- Misuses medical or technical terms, refers to studies with-

---

*Obesity & Health, editor, Frances M. Berg, Healthy Living Institute, 402 S. 14th Street, Hettinger, ND 58639, (701–567-2646).

out giving complete references, claims government approval.

- Professes to be a treatment for a wide range of ailments and nutritional deficiencies as well as for weight loss.

Program

- Promotes a medically unsupervised diet of less than 1000 calories per day.
- Diagnoses nutrient deficiencies with a computer-scored questionnaire and prescribes vitamins and supplements (rather than a balanced diet). Recommends them in excess of 100% of Recommended Dietary Allowance.
- Requires special foods purchased from the company rather than conventional foods.
- Promotes aids and devices such as: body wraps, sauna belts, electronic muscle stimulators, passive motion tables, ear stapling, aromatherapy, appetite patches, and acupuncture.
- Promotes a nutritional plan without relying on at least one author or counselor with nutrition credentials. (Nutrition educators and registered dietitians are preferred. The science of nutrition is taught only through college Home Economics and related departments.)
- Fails to state risks or recommend a medical exam.

Ingredients

- Uses unproven, bogus, or potentially dangerous ingredients such as: dinitrophenol, spirulina, amino acid supplements, glucomannan, human chorionic gonadotrophin hormone (HCG), diuretics, slimming teas, echinacea root, bee pollen, fennel, chickweed, and starch blockers. (When its review process is complete, the FDA is expected to approve only phenylpropanolamine, PPA.)
- Claims ingredients will block digestion or surround calories, starches, carbohydrates or fats, and remove them from the body.

Mystique

- Encourages reliance on a guru figure who has the "ultimate answers."
- Grants mystical properties to certain foods or ingredients.
- Bases plan on faddish ideas, such as food allergies, forbidden foods, or "magic combinations" of foods.
- Declares that the established medical community is against this discovery and refuses to accept its miraculous benefits.

Method of Availability

- Is sold by self-proclaimed health advisors or "nutritionists," often door-to-door, in "health food" stores, or a chiropractor's office.
- Distributes through hard-sell mail order advertisements, or through ads that list only an 800 number, without an address, indicating possible Postal Service action against the company.
- Demands large advance payments or long-term contracts. (Payments should be pay-as-you-go, or refundable.)
- Uses high-pressure sales tactics, one-time-only deals, or recruitment for a pyramid sales organization. Displays prominent money-back guarantee. (A common complaint against these companies is that they do not honor their guarantees.)

Questions and complaints should be directed to the State Attorney General's Office. Other agencies concerned with fraud are the FDA, FTC, Postal Service, and Better Business Bureau.

◇ Appendix B ◇

*Potential Side-effects of Very Low-calorie Diets**

Diets providing fewer than 800 calories per day have potential side effects, which may vary with the person and composition of the diet. It is strongly recommended these diets be used only in a strictly supervised hospital setting, and only when the consequences of the obesity are a greater life threat than the potential complications of the low-calorie intake.

- *Cardiac arrhythmias:* Prolonged QT interval, ventricular fibrillation, multifocal premature ventricular contractions, and atrial fibrillation have all been observed. Arrhythmias can occur suddenly, without warning, and are potentially fatal.
- *Inability to maintain long-term weight loss:* Rapid and/or repeated weight loss may slow basal metabolic rate, reducing calories needed. Lost weight may be regained quickly, and be more difficult to lose again in the future. Depression and diminished self-esteem are likely sequelae to weight regain.
- *Initiation of binge eating:* The event initiating the development of anorexia and bulimia is almost invariably severe calorie restriction.
- *Emotional changes:* VLCD's have been associated with emotional withdrawal, depression, anxiety, and irritability.

Toward Safe Weight Loss: Recommended Interim Guidelines for Adult Weight-loss Programs in Michigan, East Lansing, Mich.: Michigan Health Council, 1989, pp. 47, 48.

- *Loss of body protein:* Muscle and organ tissue is gradually lost with extreme caloric deprivation.
- *Dehydration:* VLCD's, particularly if low in carbohydrates, can induce excessive diuresis, leading to decreased blood volume, which can lead to postural hypotension. Dehydration is potentially fatal.
- *Ketosis:* VLCD's, particularly if low in carbohydrates, can cause ketosis. Ketosis is widely believed to cause euphoria and decreased appetite, although not all researchers agree. Ketosis can interfere with concentration and cause strong, unpleasant breath and body odor. In extreme cases it may lower blood pH, which can be fatal. Ketosis is hazardous for pregnant women and insulin-dependent diabetics. It can be avoided if carbohydrate and calorie levels are high enough.
- *Hypoglycemia:* VLCD's can result in excessively low levels of glucose in the blood, which may cause headaches, fatigue, inability to concentrate, sleepiness and cardiac arrhythmias.
- *Hypokalemia:* VLCD's can result in excessively low levels of potassium in the blood, which may lead to cardiac arrhythmias.
- *Hyperuricemia:* Excess uric acid levels have been caused by VLCD's. Gouty arthritis or uric acid kidney stones may be caused or exacerbated.
- *Fibrosis of vital organs:* An abnormal increase in fibrous connective tissue in the organs may occur with repeated attempts at weight loss using starvation methods.
- *Hair loss:* Hair loss is a well-documented side effect of VLCD's; usually temporary.
- *Anemia:* VLCD's have been associated with anemia, characterized by fatigue, lassitude, weakness, pallor, reduced resistance to infection, lowered exercise tolerance, and decreased attention span.
- *Re-feeding edema:* With very low carbohydrate diets, large amounts of water may be retained when carbohydrates are consumed in the re-feeding process.
- *Other documented side effects:* Among other side effects are constipation or diarrhea, headaches, nausea, dry skin, gallstones, muscle cramps, bad breath, fatigue, cold intol-

erance, menstrual irregularities, and transient skin rash.

The *Interim Guidelines* were developed for the Michigan Health Council by a broad-based task force convened at the request of the Michigan Department of Public Health in response to "potentially dangerous practices in the weight-loss industry," and written by Patricia K. Smith, MS nutrition candidate, Michigan State University, and Karen Petersmarck, MPH, RD, Project Director, Weight Loss Guidelines, Michigan Health Council. The *Interim Guidelines* are endorsed by 42 Michigan organizations and agencies and are expected to evolve into a fully endorsed, widely publicized, recognized standard of care for weight loss in Michigan.

Ordering information: *Toward Safe Weight Loss: Recommended Interim Guidelines for Adult Weight Loss Programs in Michigan* ($5.00). Michigan Health Council, 1305 Abbott Road, #102, East Lansing, MI 48823; (517) 337–1615.

◊ Appendix C ◊

Organizations for the Treatment of Eating Disorders

ANAD—National Association of Anorexia Nervosa and
  Associated Disorders.
P.O. Box 271
Highland Park, Illinois 60035
(312) 831–3438

ANRED—Anorexia Nervosa and Related Eating Disorders,
  Inc.
99 West 10th Avenue, Suite 330
Eugene, Oregon 97401
(503) 344–1144

NAAS—National Anorexic Aid Society.
550 S. Cleveland Avenue, Suite F
Westerville, Ohio 43081
(614) 895–2009

BASH—Bulimia Anorexia Self-Help, Inc.
1035 Bellevue Avenue, Suite 104
St. Louis, Missouri 63117
(314) 567–4080 or (314) 991–BASH

American Anorexia/Bulimia Association, Inc.
133 Cedar Lane
Teaneck, New Jersey 07666
(201) 836–1800

◇ Appendix D ◇

Menu Ideas

The following menu ideas have been prepared by Lisa Harris, RD, a licensed Nutrition Consultant. While no recipes are provided, preparation ideas are included. We have looked for simplicity and practicality in our menus.

Most of the items suggested are commercially available. Every nutritional standard is met and variety is encouraged. The calorie amounts at the top of the meal lists are the whole-day allotments.

In preparation, remember to keep your fat content as low as possible, and try to adapt some of your family's favorite recipes so you can eat with them as well. Remember, if it's good for you, it's good for them.

When serving canned fruit, rinsing is recommended unless it comes packed in light syrup or in fruit juice.

Bon Appetit!

BREAKFAST	1400	1600	1800	2000
Bread	2	2	3	3
Meat*	0–1	0–1	0–1	0–1
Fruit	1	1	1	1
Milk	1	1	1	1
Fat†	0–1	0–1	0–1	0–1
LUNCH				
Bread	2	3	3	3
Meat	2	3	3	3
Vegetable	1	1	1	1
Fruit	1	1	2	2
Milk	1	1	1	1
Fat	0–1	1	1	2
DINNER				
Bread	3	3	3	3
Meat	3	3	4	4
Vegetable	1	1	1	2
Fruit	1	1	1	2
Milk	1	1	1	1
Fat	0–1	1	1	2

---

*On days when one protein is used at breakfast, delete one serving of protein from dinner.
†Adjust fat servings per totals allowed each day.

Breakfast	1400	1600	1800	2000
#1				
wheat-flake cereal	¾ c	¾ c	1½ c	1½ c
whole wheat toast	1 slice	1 slice	1 slice	1 slice
orange juice	½ c	½ c	½ c	½ c
milk, skim	1 c	1 c	1 c	1 c
margarine	1 tsp	1 tsp	1 tsp	1 tsp
#2				
oatmeal, cooked with 1 tsp brown sugar	1 c	1 c	1½ c	1½ c
raisins	2 tbsp	2 tbsp	2 tbsp	2 tbsp
milk, skim	1 c	1 c	1 c	1 c
#3				
whole wheat English muffin	1	1	1½	1½
peanut butter	1 tbsp	1 tbsp	1 tbsp	1 tbsp
sliced apple w/cinnamon	1	1	1	1
milk, skim	1 c	1 c	1 c	1 c
#4				
whole wheat English muffin	1	1	1½	1½
scrambled egg	1	1	1	1
apple juice	½ c	½ c	½ c	½ c
milk, skim	1 c	1 c	1 c	1 c
margarine	1 tsp	1 tsp	1 tsp	1 tsp
#5				
cold cereal	1½ c	1½ c	1½ c	1½ c
whole wheat toast	0	0	1 slice	1 slice
banana	½	½	½	½
milk, skim	1 c	1 c	1 c	1 c
margarine	0	0	1 tsp	1 tsp
#6				
hot cereal, cooked with 1 tsp sugar & cinnamon	1 c	1 c	1 c	1 c
raisin toast, unfrosted	0	0	1 slice	1 slice
orange juice	½ c	½ c	½ c	½ c
milk, skim	1 c	1 c	1 c	1 c
margarine	0	0	1 tsp	1 tsp
#7				
Grape Nuts™	6 tbsp	6 tbsp	6 tbsp	6 tbsp
raisin toast, unfrosted	0	0	1 slice	1 slice

banana	½	½	½	½
vanilla yogurt, nonfat	½ c	½ c	½ c	½ c
milk, skim	½ c	½ c	½ c	½ c
margarine	0	0	1 tsp	1 tsp

#8

French toast:	2 slices	2 slices	3 slices	3 slices
whole wheat bread dipped in mixture of:				
egg	1	1	1	1
milk, skim	2 tbsp	2 tbsp	2 tbsp	2 tbsp
cinnamon,				
honey or syrup (optional)	1 tbsp	1 tbsp	1 tbsp	1 tbsp
applesauce	½ c	½ c	½ c	½ c
milk, skim	¾ c	¾ c	¾ c	¾ c

#9

homemade "Danish":				
English muffin	1	1	1½	1½
ricotta cheese	¼ c	¼ c	¼ c	¼ c
applesauce	½ c	½ c	½ c	½ c
(sprinkle w/cinnamon and heat in toaster oven until cheese is melted)				
milk, skim	1 c	1 c	1 c	1 c

#10

whole wheat toast	2 slices	2 slices	2 slices	2 slices
flake cereal	0	0	¾ c	¾ c
poached egg	1	1	1	1
pineapple juice	½ c	½ c	½ c	½ c
milk, skim	1 c	1 c	1 c	1 c
margarine	1 tsp	1 tsp	1 tsp	1 tsp

#11

waffle, 4½" square	2	2	3	3
syrup, optional	1 tbsp	1 tbsp	1 tbsp	1 tbsp
applesauce	½ c	½ c	½ c	½ c
milk, skim	1 c	1 c	1 c	1 c
margarine	1 tsp	1 tsp	1 tsp	1 tsp

#12

graham crackers, 2½" square	6 each	6 each	6 each	6 each
wheat-flake cereal	0	0	¾ c	¾ c
cottage cheese, lowfat	¼ c	¼ c	¼ c	¼ c
cantaloupe	⅓ melon	⅓ melon	⅓ melon	⅓ melon
milk, skim	1 c	1 c	1 c	1 c

#13

muffin, oat bran or fruit	1 med	1 med	1 lg	1 lg
banana	½	½	½	½
milk, skim	1 c	1 c	1 c	1 c

#14

breakfast bar*, no more than 150 calories and 30% fat	1	1	2	2
apple juice	½ c	½ c	½ c	½ c
milk, skim	1 c	1 c	1 c	1 c

#15

instant breakfast mix* with skim milk	1 c	1 c	1 c	1 c
banana	½	½	½	½
whole wheat toast	0	0	1	1
margarine	0	0	1 tsp	1 tsp

---

*Commercial products found in the breakfast food section of the supermarket.

Lunch	1400	1600	1800	2000
#1				
tuna sandwich with:				
whole wheat bread	2 slices	2 slices	2 slices	2 slices
tuna, water-packed	½ c	¾ c	¾ c	¾ c
mayonnaise, reduced calorie,	1 tbsp	1 tbsp	1 tbsp	2 tbsp
chopped celery and onions				
whole wheat crackers, no fat added	0	3	3	3
celery sticks	½ c	½ c	½ c	½ c
apple	1 small	1 small	1 large	1 large
milk, skim	1 c	1 c	1 c	1 c
#2				
chili with beans	1 c	1 c	1 c	1 c
grated lowfat cheese	0	1 oz	1 oz	1 oz
whole wheat roll	0	1	1	1
carrot sticks	½ c	½ c	½ c	½ c
banana	½	½	1	1
milk, skim	1 c	1 c	1 c	1 c
#3				
whole wheat pita	1	1	1	1
with turkey, chopped	2 oz	3 oz	3 oz	3 oz
lettuce	1 leaf	1 leaf	1 leaf	1 leaf
raisins	0	0	2 tbsp	2 tbsp
mayo, reduced calorie	1 tbsp	1 tbsp	1 tbsp	2 tbsp
grapes	15	15	15	15
animal crackers	0	8	8	8
milk, skim	1 c	1 c	1 c	1 c
#4				
submarine sandwich:				
small roll	1	1	1	1
beef, lean	½ oz	½ oz	½ oz	½ oz
turkey	½ oz	1 oz	1 oz	1 oz
ham, lean	½ oz	1 oz	1 oz	1 oz
cheese	½ oz	½ oz	½ oz	½ oz
(slice meats and cheese very thin)				
mayo, reduced calorie	1 tbsp	1 tbsp	1 tbsp	1 tbsp
avocado	0	0	0	⅛
mustard				
pretzels	0	¾ oz	¾ oz	¾ oz
carrot sticks	½ c	½ c	½ c	½ c

orange, sliced	1	1	1	1
apple, sliced	0	0	1	1
milk, skim	1 c	1 c	1 c	1 c

#5

bagel	1	1	1	1
fruit "ambrosia":				
lowfat cottage cheese	½ c	¾ c	¾ c	¾ c
lowfat yogurt,	¼ c	¼ c	¼ c	¼ c
fruit-flavored				
peaches, diced	¼ c	¼ c	½ c	½ c
topped with Grape Nuts™	0	3 tbsp	3 tbsp	3 tbsp
salad	½ c	½ c	½ c	½ c
diet salad dressing	2 tbsp	2 tbsp	2 tbsp	2 tbsp
milk, skim	1 c	1 c	1 c	1 c

#6

vegetable soup	1 c	1 c	1 c	1 c
chicken salad sandwich:				
whole wheat bread	1 slice	2 slices	2 slices	2 slices
chicken, chopped	2 oz	3 oz	3 oz	3 oz
diet salad dressing	2 tbsp	2 tbsp	2 tbsp	4 tbsp
tomato	2 slices	2 slices	2 slices	2 slices
lettuce	1 leaf	1 leaf	1 leaf	1 leaf
pear, fresh	1 small	1 small	1 large	1 large
milk, skim	1 c	1 c	1 c	1 c

#7

baked chicken	2 oz	3 oz	3 oz	3 oz
baked beans	½ c	½ c	½ c	½ c
salad	½ c	½ c	½ c	½ c
diet salad dressing	2 tbsp	2 tbsp	2 tbsp	2 tbsp
whole wheat roll	0	1	1	1
banana	½	½	1	1
milk, skim	1 c	1 c	1 c	1 c
margarine	0	1 tsp	1 tsp	1 tsp

#8

spaghetti (cooked noodles)	1 c	1 c	1 c	1 c
with: meatballs	1 oz	2 oz	2 oz	2 oz
sauce	½ c	½ c	½ c	½ c
parmesan cheese	2 tbsp	2 tbsp	2 tbsp	2 tbsp
bread sticks, 4" long	0	2	2	2
spinach	½ c	½ c	½ c	½ c
applesauce	½ c	½ c	1 c	1 c
milk, skim	1 c	1 c	1 c	1 c
margarine	0	1 tsp	1 tsp	2 tsp

#9

baked potato	1 large	1 large	1 large	1 large
topped with:				
taco-flavored beef	2 oz	2 oz	2 oz	2 oz
shredded lowfat cheese	0	1 oz	1 oz	1 oz
sour cream	0	2 tbsp	2 tbsp	2 tbsp
margarine	0	0	0	1 tsp
green beans	½ c	½ c	½ c	½ c
Rye-Krisp™	0	4	4	4
pineapple, canned	⅓ c	⅓ c	⅔ c	⅔ c
milk, skim	1 c	1 c	1 c	1 c

#10

hamburger patty	3 oz	3 oz	4 oz	4 oz
with cheese	0	1 oz	1 oz	1 oz
pickles, catsup, mustard				
French fries	0	10 each	10 each	10 each
salad	½ c	½ c	½ c	½ c
diet salad dressing	2 tbsp	2 tbsp	2 tbsp	2 tbsp
apple	1 small	1 small	1 large	1 large
milk, skim	1 c	1 c	1 c	1 c

#11

pizza, cheese, ¼ of a 10″ pizza	1 slice	1 slice	2 slices	2 slices
with: lean Canadian	1 oz	2 oz	1 oz	1 oz
bacon				
bread sticks, 4″ long	0	2	1	1
salad	½ c	½ c	½ c	½ c
diet salad dressing	2 tbsp	2 tbsp	2 tbsp	2 tbsp
peach, fresh	1 small	1 small	1 large	1 large
milk, skim	1 c	1 c	½ c	½ c

#12

peanut butter & jelly sandwich:				
whole wheat bread	2 slices	2 slices	2 slices	2 slices
peanut butter	2 tbsp	2 tbsp	2 tbsp	2 tbsp
jelly	1 tbsp	1 tbsp	1 tbsp	1 tbsp
string cheese	0	1 oz	1 oz	1 oz
yogurt, lemon-flavored, nonfat	1 c	1 c	1 c	1 c
carrot sticks	½ c	½ c	½ c	½ c
graham crackers	0	3	3	3
apple juice	½ c	½ c	1 c	1 c
olives	0	5 large	5 large	10 large

#13
soft taco with:				
ground beef, lean	2 oz	2 oz	2 oz	2 oz
grated cheese	0	1 oz	1 oz	1 oz
lettuce & tomato	½ c	½ c	½ c	½ c
flour tortilla	1	1	1	1
refried beans	⅓ c	⅔ c	⅔ c	⅔ c
pears, canned	2 halves	2 halves	4 halves	4 halves
milk, skim	1 c	1 c	1 c	1 c

#14
frozen lowfat dinner (less than 300 calories)	1	1	1	1
salad	½ c	½ c	½ c	½ c
diet salad dressing	2 tbsp	2 tbsp	2 tbsp	2 tbsp
apple, sliced	0	0	1	1
milk, skim	1 c	1 c	1 c	1 c
(save for snack:)				
cheese	0	1 oz	1 oz	1 oz
saltines	0	6	6	6

Dinner	1400	1600	1800	2000
#1				
savory chicken breast	3 oz	3 oz	4 oz	4 oz
(marinate in low-cal Italian dressing)				
wild rice, cooked	⅔ c	⅔ c	⅔ c	⅔ c
whole wheat roll	1 small	1 small	1 small	1 small
broccoli	½ c	½ c	½ c	1 c
peaches, canned	½ c	½ c	½ c	1 c
milk, skim	1 c	1 c	1 c	1 c
margarine	1 tsp	1 tsp	1 tsp	2 tsp
#2				
baked halibut w/lemon	3 oz	3 oz	4 oz	4 oz
new potatoes	6 oz	6 oz	6 oz	6 oz
cooked w/parsley and				
margarine	1 tsp	1 tsp	1 tsp	2 tsp
baked beans	¼ c	¼ c	¼ c	¼ c
salad	½ c	½ c	½ c	1 c
diet salad dressing	2 tbsp	2 tbsp	2 tbsp	2 tbsp
fruit cocktail	½ c	½ c	½ c	1 c
milk, skim	1 c	1 c	1 c	1 c
#3				
spaghetti (cooked noodles)	1 c	1 c	1 c	1 c
with:				
ground beef	2 oz	2 oz	2 oz	2 oz
sauce	· ½ c	½ c	½ c	½ c
parmesan cheese	2 tbsp	2 tbsp	4 tbsp	4 tbsp
French bread	1 slice	1 slice	1 slice	1 slice
zucchini	½ c	½ c	½ c	1 c
frozen grapes	15 small	15 small	15 small	15 small
honeydew melon	0	0	0	1 c
milk, skim	1 c	1 c	1 c	1 c
margarine	1 tsp	1 tsp	1 tsp	2 tsp
#4				
BBQ flank steak	3 oz	3 oz	4 oz	4 oz
corn on the cob, 6″	1	1	1	1
noodles, cooked	1 c	1 c	1 c	1 c
seasoned w/parsley				
& margarine	1 tsp	1 tsp	1 tsp	2 tsp
green beans	½ c	½ c	½ c	1 c
strawberries	1¼ c	1¼ c	1¼ c	1¼ c
kiwi, slices	0	0	0	1
milk, skim	1 c	1 c	1 c	1 c

#5

Italian chicken:				
breast	3 oz	3 oz	4 oz	4 oz
cooked in stewed	½ c	½ c	½ c	1 c
tomatoes				
(seasoned w/Italian seasoning, garlic & onion powder)				
shell pasta, cooked	1 c	1 c	1 c	1 c
peas	½ c	½ c	½ c	½ c
apple, sliced	1	1	1	1
orange, sliced	0	0	0	1
milk, skim	1 c	1 c	1 c	1 c
margarine	1 tsp	1 tsp	1 tsp	2 tsp

#6

turkey, sliced	3 oz	3 oz	4 oz	4 oz
dressing	½ c	½ c	½ c	½ c
yams	⅓ c	⅓ c	⅓ c	⅓ c
green beans	½ c	½ c	½ c	1 c
applesauce w/cinnamon	½ c	½ c	½ c	1 c
milk, skim	1 c	1 c	1 c	1 c
margarine	0	0	0	1 tsp

#7

shrimp, steamed	6 oz	6 oz	8 oz	8 oz
black beans, cooked	⅓ c	⅓ c	⅓ c	⅓ c
(seasoned w/onions, garlic powder, mushrooms)				
brown rice, cooked	⅔ c	⅔ c	⅔ c	⅔ c
sliced tomatoes	3 slices	3 slices	3 slices	6 slices
diet gelatin w/ diced pears	½ c	½ c	½ c	1 c
milk, skim	1 c	1 c	1 c	1 c
margarine	1 tsp	1 tsp	1 tsp	2 tsp

#8

pork chops, broiled (trim fat)	3 oz	3 oz	4 oz	4 oz
potatoes, mashed	½ c	½ c	½ c	½ c
dinner roll	1 large	1 large	1 large	1 large
spinach	½ c	½ c	½ c	1 c
applesauce	½ c	½ c	½ c	½ c
w/raisins	0	0	0	2 tbsp
milk, skim	1 c	1 c	1 c	1 c
margarine	1 tsp	1 tsp	1 tsp	2 tsp

#9
beef stew (make in crock pot
with no added fat)

lean beef	3 oz	3 oz	4 oz	4 oz
potatoes, chopped	1 small	1 small	1 small	1 small
carrots	½ c	½ c	½ c	½ c
peas	½ c	½ c	½ c	½ c
biscuit	1	1	1	1
peaches, canned	2 halves	2 halves	2 halves	4 halves
milk, skim	1 c	1 c	1 c	1 c
margarine	0	0	0	1 tsp

#10

ham, lean	3 oz	3 oz	4 oz	4 oz
cornbread, 2″ sq.	1	1	1	1
sweet potato	⅔ c	⅔ c	⅔ c	⅔ c
salad	½ c	½ c	½ c	1 c
diet salad dressing	2 tbsp	2 tbsp	2 tbsp	2 tbsp
fruit cocktail	½ c	½ c	½ c	1 c
milk, skim	1 c	1 c	1 c	1 c
margarine	0	0	0	1 tsp

#11

broiled swordfish	3 oz	3 oz	4 oz	4 oz
baked potato	1 large	1 large	1 large	1 large
w/chives & sour cream	2 tbsp	2 tbsp	2 tbsp	2 tbsp
salad	½ c	½ c	½ c	1 c
diet salad dressing	2 tbsp	2 tbsp	2 tbsp	2 tbsp
sherbet	¼ c	¼ c	¼ c	¼ c
raspberries	½ c	½ c	½ c	1 c
(save for snack:)				
banana	¼	¼	¼	½
milk, skim	1 c	1 c	1 c	1 c

#12

hamburger patty	3 oz	3 oz	4 oz	4 oz
whole wheat bun	1	1	1	1
lettuce & tomato,				
reduced calorie mayo	1 tbsp	1 tbsp	1 tbsp	2 tbsp
mustard & catsup				
baked beans	¼ c	¼ c	¼ c	¼ c
watermelon cubes	1¼ c	1¼ c	1¼ c	1¼ c
cantaloupe	0	0	0	⅓ melon
milk, skim	1 c	1 c	1 c	1 c

#13

filet of sole, broiled, with lemon & herbs	3 oz	3 oz	4 oz	4 oz
baked potato (wedges)	1 small	1 small	1 small	1 small
broccoli	½ c	½ c	½ c	1 c
peach slices	½ c	½ c	½ c	1 c
milk, skim	1 c	1 c	1 c	1 c
margarine	1 tsp	1 tsp	1 tsp	2 tsp
angel food cake, ½ piece	1	1	1	1

#14

seasoned chicken, baked w/choice of spices	3 oz	3 oz	4 oz	4 oz
mashed potatoes	½ c	½ c	½ c	½ c
corn	½ c	½ c	½ c	½ c
salad	½ c	½ c	½ c	1 c
diet salad dressing	2 tbsp	2 tbsp	2 tbsp	2 tbsp
fruit cocktail	½ c	½ c	½ c	1 c
milk, skim	1 c	1 c	1 c	1 c
margarine	1 tsp	1 tsp	1 tsp	2 tsp
animal crackers	8	8	8	8

◇ Appendix E ◇

Recommended Reading

The following list is based in part on reviews from *The Current Diet Review*, Lisa Harris, R.D., a clinical and consulting nutitionist and editor. These books should be available through your local bookstore. If not, inquire about ordering them.

Bailey, Covert. *The Fit or Fat Target Diet*, (Houghton Mufflin Co. 1984).

Brody, Jane. *Jane Brody's Good Food Book: Living the High-Carbohydrate Way*, (W.W. Norton and Company, 1985).

Callaway, C. Wayne, M.D. and Catherine Whitney. *The Callaway Diet: Successful Permanent Weight Control for Starvers, Stuffers, and Skippers*, (Bantam Books).

Conor, Sonja L. and William E. *The New American Diet*, (Simon and Schuster, 1986).

Edwards, Sally. *The Equilibrium Plan*, (Arbor House, 1987).

Ferguson, James M., M.D. *Habits, Not Diets: The Secret to Lifetime Weight Control*, (Bull Publishing Company).

Franz, Marion J. R., R.D., M.S. *Exchanges for All Occasions*, (The Diabetes Center, Inc.).

Jennings-Sauer, Cherly. *Living Lean by Choosing More*, (Taylor Publishing Company, 1989).

Lamb, Lawrence E. *The Weighting Game*, (Lyle Stuart, Inc., 1988).

Leveille, Gilbert. *The Setpoint Diet*, (Ballentine Books, 1985).

Smith, Pamela, M., R.D. *The Food Trap*, (Creation House).

Tribole, Evelyn. *Eating on the Run*, (Life Enhancement Publications, 1987).

Special Thanks

To my family, who have been most supportive during the tough days it has taken to live, research, and write this material.

To my friends, who have been especially patient and unselfishly given of their time to listen to one-sided conversations and read drafts of this work at different stages of its progress. The Neva Coyle Ministries board of directors has been supportive and encouraging—while keeping me accountable. Thanks to Glen, Terry, Marieta, and Chuck.

And, very special thanks to David Hazard, a gifted editor who, like a skillful cosmetic surgeon, has made this project better without leaving scars on either the book or me.

Books by Neva Coyle:

Free To Be Thin, w/Marie Chapian, a successful weight-loss plan which links learning how to eat with how to live

Free to Dream, biblical insights on wishes, dreams, and goals

Overcoming the Dieting Dilemma faces the problem of the dieter who has done everything right but without seeing the desired results.

There's More To Being Thin Than Being Thin, w/Marie Chapian, focusing on the valuable lessons learned on the *journey* to being thin

Slimming Down and Growing Up, w/Marie Chapian, applying the "Free To Be Thin" principles to kids

Living Free, her personal testimony

Daily Thoughts on Living Free, a devotional

Scriptures for Living Free, a counter-top display book of Scriptures to accompany the devotional

Free To Be Thin Cookbook, a collection of tasty, nutritious recipes complete with the calorie content of each

Free To Be Thin Leader's Kit, a step-by-step guide for organizing and leading an Overeaters Victorious group, including five cassette tapes of instruction

Free To Be Thin Daily Planner, a three-month planner for recording daily thoughts, activities and calorie intake

Getting Your Family On Your Side, how a dieter's family and close friends influence weight-management's successes and failures